Register Now for
to Your I

SPRINGER PUBLISHING COMPANY

CONNECT™

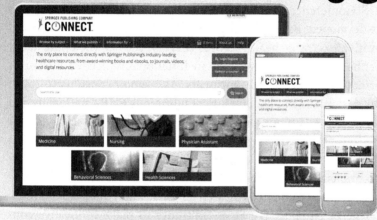

Your print purchase of *Application of Nursing Informatics* **includes online access to the contents of your book**—increasing accessibility, portability, and searchability!

Access today at:

**http://connect.springerpub.com/content/book/978-0-8261-4122-4
or scan the QR code at the right with your smartphone
and enter the access code below.**

H5F5FGDE

*Scan here for
quick access.*

If you are experiencing problems accessing the digital component of this product, please contact our customer service department at cs@springerpub.com

The online access with your print purchase is available at the publisher's discretion and may be removed at any time without notice.

Publisher's Note: New and used products purchased from third-party sellers are not guaranteed for quality, authenticity, or access to any included digital components.

SPRINGER PUBLISHING COMPANY

View all our products at springerpub.com

Carolyn Sipes, PhD, CNS, APRN, RN-BC, PMP, NEA-BC, FAAN, is a professor of nursing informatics and leadership at the graduate masters and doctoral levels, previously at Chamberlain University and currently at Walden University. Dr. Sipes has over 35 years of nursing experience, has served in leadership positions, and is a teaching/learning innovator. Her clinical and subsequent teaching practice has been informed and enhanced by her ongoing research. Dr. Sipes was a pioneer in various areas of AIDS research. As the principal investigator (PI) she presented research at the XIV International AIDS Conference in Barcelona on a medication compliance and tolerability tool that she developed. Based on her years of experience in the creation and design of the first innovative electronic health records (EHRs), she had the opportunity to contribute to their enhancement by filling gaps in functionality needed by nurses but overlooked by information technology departments. As a senior consultant/project manager/director for the design and implementation of numerous EHRs, nationally and internationally, Dr. Sipes developed unique informatics competency-skill assessments for all clinical departments. These were used as pre/posttraining assessments in preparation for EHR implementation and provided data organizations used to identify the need for further training prior to implementation. She has authored numerous publications and informatics competencies, and has presented research nationally and internationally.

At Chamberlain College of Nursing, Dr. Sipes continues to make innovative contributions in the specialty of nursing informatics as well as other education endeavors such as master instruction, research, and technology. Dr. Sipes has published and presented numerous articles and scholarly papers on nursing informatics, nationally and internationally, including the World CIST conference in Lisbon, Portugal, and the World Nursing Informatics Conference, Geneva, and the 4th International Congress on Nursing, Valencia. She recently contributed chapters to the *Handbook of Informatics for Nurses and Healthcare Professionals* (2018), a nursing informatics book, and *Project Management for the Advance Practice Nurse,* which included tool development (2016). Currently, she is the PI on a research project that is assessing competency levels in graduate faculty with the goal of providing support to faculty who need to improve their informatics skills. Her clinical, leadership, and nursing-education experience provide a wealth of knowledge and innovative skill that Dr. Sipes continues to apply to her nursing practice and her research in informatics. She is a fellow of the American Academy of Nursing.

APPLICATION OF NURSING INFORMATICS

Competencies, Skills, Decision-Making

Carolyn Sipes, PhD, CNS, APRN, RN-BC, PMP, NEA-BC, FAAN

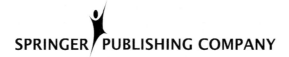
SPRINGER PUBLISHING COMPANY

Copyright © 2019 Springer Publishing Company, LLC

All rights reserved.

No part of this publication may be reproduced, stored in a retrieval system, or transmitted in any form or by any means, electronic, mechanical, photocopying, recording, or otherwise, without the prior permission of Springer Publishing Company, LLC, or authorization through payment of the appropriate fees to the Copyright Clearance Center, Inc., 222 Rosewood Drive, Danvers, MA 01923, 978-750-8400, fax 978-646-8600, info@copyright.com or on the Web at www.copyright.com.

Springer Publishing Company, LLC
11 West 42nd Street
New York, NY 10036
www.springerpub.com

Acquisitions Editor: Joseph Morita
Compositor: S4Carlisle Publishing Services

ISBN: 978-0-8261-4119-4
ebook ISBN: 978-0-8261-4122-4
Instructor's Manual: 978-0-8261-4158-3
Instructor's PowerPoints: 978-0-8261-4148-4

Instructor's Materials: Qualified instructors may request supplements by emailing textbook@springerpub.com.

19 20 21 22 23 / 5 4 3 2 1

The author and the publisher of this Work have made every effort to use sources believed to be reliable to provide information that is accurate and compatible with the standards generally accepted at the time of publication. Because medical science is continually advancing, our knowledge base continues to expand. Therefore, as new information becomes available, changes in procedures become necessary. We recommend that the reader always consult current research and specific institutional policies before performing any clinical procedure. The author and publisher shall not be liable for any special, consequential, or exemplary damages resulting, in whole or in part, from the readers' use of, or reliance on, the information contained in this book. The publisher has no responsibility for the persistence or accuracy of URLs for external or third-party Internet websites referred to in this publication and does not guarantee that any content on such websites is, or will remain, accurate or appropriate.

Library of Congress Cataloging-in-Publication Data
Names: Sipes, Carolyn, editor.
Title: Application of nursing informatics:
   competencies, skills, decision-making / [edited by] Carolyn Sipes.
Description: New York : Springer Publishing Company, [2019] | Includes
   bibliographical references and index.
Identifiers: LCCN 2018041930| ISBN 9780826141194 | ISBN 9780826141583
   (instructors manual) | ISBN 9780826141224 (ebook) | ISBN 9780826141484
   (instructors PowerPoints)
Subjects: | MESH: Medical Informatics Applications | Nursing Informatics
Classification: LCC R858 | NLM WY 26.5 | DDC 610.285--dc23 LC record available at
https://lccn.loc.gov/2018041930

Contact us to receive discount rates on bulk purchases.
We can also customize our books to meet your needs.
For more information please contact: sales@springerpub.com

Publisher's Note: New and used products purchased from third-party sellers are not guaranteed for quality, authenticity, or access to any included digital components.

Printed in the United States of America.

CONTENTS

CONTRIBUTORS

Lisa M. Blair, PhD, RNC-NIC   Research Associate, School of Nursing, University of Virginia, Charlottesville, Virginia

Christine S. Gipson, PhD, RN, CNE   Assistant Professor, RN–BSN Coordinator, The University of Texas at Tyler, Tyler, Texas

Lynda Hardy, PhD, RN, FAAN   Director, Data Science and Discovery, Associate Professor, College of Nursing, Ohio State University, Columbus, Ohio

Toni Hebda, PhD, MNEd, MSIS, RN-C   Professor, MSN Program, Chamberlain College of Nursing, Downers Grove, Illinois

Melinda Hermanns, PhD, RN-BC, CNE, PH/FCN   Associate Professor, MSN Program Director, The University of Texas at Tyler, Tyler, Texas

Taryn Hill, PhD, RN   Dean of Academic Affairs, Chamberlain College of Nursing, Columbus, Ohio

Kathleen Hunter, PhD, RN-BC, CNE, FAAN   Professor, MSN Program, Chamberlain College of Nursing, Downers Grove, Illinois

Cheryl D. Parker, PhD, MSN, RN-BC, CNE, FHIMSS   Clinical Assistant Professor, College of Nursing and Health Sciences, The University of Texas at Tyler, Tyler, Texas

Carolyn Sipes, PhD, CNS, APRN, RN-BC, PMP, NEA-BC, FAAN   Professor, MSN program, Chamberlain College of Nursing, Downers Grove, Illinois; DNP PhD Program, Walden University, Minneapolis, Minnesota

James Sipes, BEE, MSEE   Electrical Engineer, Ohio State University, Columbus, Ohio

Karen West, MSN RN   Virtual Learning Experiences, Faculty Support Specialist, MSN Program, Chamberlain College of Nursing, Downers Grove, Illinois

PREFACE

Why is understanding nursing informatics (NI) important? Why do we, as nurses, need to develop and use NI skills, knowledge, and competencies in clinical practice? Examining the research that follows is the best way to explain this need for informatics.

In researching nursing informatics, the Student Working Group of the International Medical Informatics Association Nursing Informatics Special Interest Group (IMIA NISIG) developed and distributed an international survey of current and future trends in NI (Topaz et al., 2016). The survey was developed based on current literature concerned with NI trends and was translated into six languages. Respondents were from 31 different countries in Asia, Africa, North and Central America, South America, Europe, and Australia. The results of responses to the survey question: "What should be done (at a country or organizational level) to advance nursing informatics in the next 5–10 years?" Participants' ($N = 272$) responses were grouped according to five key themes: (a) education and training, (b) research, (c) practice, (d) visibility, and (e) collaboration and integration (Topaz et al., 2016).

Similar findings also support the need for nurses to develop NI competencies, knowledge, and skills as noted in the IMIA NSIG study. In all, 373 responses, which came from 44 different countries, were analyzed. The responses identified the top 10 NI trends: big-data science, standardized terminologies (clinical evaluation/implementation), education and competencies, clinical decision support, mobile health, usability, patient safety, data exchange and interoperability, patient engagement, and clinical quality measures (Peltonen et al., 2016).

Many of these topics are covered in this book; descriptions are enhanced with examples and case scenarios based on real-life applications. Also included are critical thinking challenges and decision-making activities to enhance skills learned.

The idea for this book came from Janet Weber, EdD, Professor Emerita of Nursing at Southeast Missouri State University. After teaching for 37 years, Dr. Weber proposed a textbook series for RN–BSN and graduate nurses. This book on the basics of NI *is part of her vision.*

Dr. Weber's request came to me, a professor in NI at Chamberlain College of Nursing. I am certified in NI, have practiced and published extensively—both nationally and internationally—on NI, and authored *Project Management for the Advanced Practice Nurse* for Springer Publishing Company.

The organizing framework for this book comes from the American Nurses Association (ANA; 2015) book *Nursing Informatics: Scope and Standards of Practice*, plus years of industry practice experience in data and data management, technology, and designing and implementing electronic health records nationally and internationally, as well as faculty expertise in these areas. Mandates by national organizations, such as the Institute of Medicine (IOM) and the ANA, indicate that nurses must possess more technology skills to meet ever-evolving workforce demands in high-tech healthcare practice environments. This book was designed to provide a basic understanding of these technology requirements, using the NI knowledge and skills needed in today's practice workforce as well as the basic considerations necessary for professional development and lifelong learning. As such, it is a collaboration produced by a community of NI faculty, technology experts, and informatics nurse specialist (INS) practitioners.

■ Organization

The book is organized into seven parts: Foundations of Nursing Informatics; Nursing Informatics: Essential Computer Concepts; Nursing Informatics: Clinical Applications; Nursing Informatics: Data Applications; Nursing Informatics: Managing Quality, Assessment, and Evaluation; Nursing Informatics: Ethics, Privacy, and Security; and Nursing Informatics: Professional Development and Advancement. An overview of these sections and the chapters within each section follows.

NI is introduced in Chapter 1 and is tied to other concepts in each of the subsequent chapters. Throughout the volume, questions are posed to readers to encourage consideration of real-life applications, critical thinking, and decision-making based on the content.

Part I: Foundations of Nursing Informatics

This section provides a foundation of NI and explains its rapid evolution and importance as well as guiding principles mandated by national organizations. It includes the knowledge and skill expectations the healthcare industry regards as basic to clinical practice in today's high-tech healthcare environment.

- Chapter 1: Nursing Informatics: Definition, Evolution, Guiding Principles, Expectations
- Chapter 2: Nursing Informatics: Roles, Professional Organizations, and Theories

Part II: Nursing Informatics: Essential Computer Concepts

This section provides the basics to understating the primary tool used by nurses in today's clinical practice—the computer—as well as other technology and software needed in nursing practice. Explanations of what the different components are, why they are important, how they function, and applications to practice are provided. Case scenarios and critical thinking questions and activities are included to engage the reader and enhance understanding of concepts.

- Chapter 3: Nursing Informatics: First Things First—Hardware
- Chapter 4: Nursing Informatics: First Things First—Software

Part III: Nursing Informatics: Clinical Applications

This section takes the reader further into clinical applications of NI as it investigates NI's general, everyday use in project management as correlated with the nursing process, applications of NI and computer concepts used in research, as well as how NI and technology work together to support education. It provides descriptions of the different learning environments and the roles they play in dynamic healthcare educational systems and defines current needed informatics skills to support information literacy and educational effectiveness.

- Chapter 5: Nursing Informatics: Project Management
- Chapter 6: Nursing Informatics: Research Applications
- Chapter 7: Nursing Informatics: Applications to Support Educational Initiatives

Part IV: Nursing Informatics: Data Applications

The section addresses data standardization applications, how to capture data, big data applications and how they inform practice and tie together NI concepts, knowledge, and skills.

- Chapter 8: Data Standardization Applications—Capturing Data
- Chapter 9: Nursing Informatics: Big Data Applications to Inform Practice

Part V: Nursing Informatics: Managing Quality, Assessment, and Evaluation

This section discusses how using technology and NI skills is necessary to understanding and maintaining the quality of data in a variety of settings. It provides an overview of the connection among data, information, knowledge, and wisdom; offers definitions for *quality* and *data quality*; and the criteria used for quality data and information during input, storage, and at retrieval, display, and printing. The chapter concludes with a review of competencies needed by the baccalaureate-prepared nurse in today's healthcare setting to recognize data quality, problems with data quality, and corrective measures. It further discusses assessment and how to evaluate outcomes using technology.

- Chapter 10: Nursing Informatics: Maintaining Quality of Data and Information
- Chapter 11: Assessment and Evaluating Outcomes

Part VI: Nursing Informatics: Ethics, Privacy, and Security

This section examines the ethics of privacy and information, security and security issues, and other issues related to the use (or incorrect use) of technology; other technology challenges that occur in today's high-tech healthcare industry are considered.

- Chapter 12: Nursing Informatics: Ethics, Privacy, Security, Other Technology Challenges

Part VII: Nursing Informatics: Professional Development and Advancement

A most important skill is to understand the value of continuing one's education and to be able tand move forward with one's own education and practice, especially in today's high-tech healthcare environment. The chapter in this section provides examples of how to use technology software to create scholarly works for school, clinical practice, and publications.

- Chapter 13: Nursing Informatics: Lifelong Learning—Advancing Your Own Education

Carolyn Sipes

References

American Nurses Association. (2015). *Nursing informatics: Scope and standards of practice* (2nd ed.). Silver Spring, MD: Author.

Peltonen, L. M., Topaz, M., Ronquillo, C., Pruinelli, L., Sarmiento, R. F., Badger, M. K., … Alhuwail, D. (2016). Nursing informatics research priorities for the future: Recommendations from an international survey. *Studies in Health Technology and Informatics, 225*, 222–226.

Topaz, M., Ronquillo, C., Peltonen, L. M., Pruinelli, L., Sarmiento, R. F., Badger, M. K., … Alhuwail, D. (2016). Advancing nursing informatics in the next decade: Recommendations from an international survey. *Studies in Health Technology and Informatics, 225,*123–127.

ACKNOWLEDGMENTS

This book was made possible by individuals dedicated to sharing their knowledge and expertise in the specialty of nursing informatics. Their commitment of time and effort comes from a desire to expand others' knowledge and to provide support in this fast-moving, quickly evolving, new nursing specialty. I am thankful for the support and contributions of peer faculty at Chamberlain College of Nursing made possible by our nursing informatics research team, which includes Toni Hebda, PhD, MNEd, MSIS, RN-C; Kathleen Hunter, PhD, RN-BC, CNE, FAAN; Taryn Hill, PhD, RN; Dee McGonigle, PhD, RN, CNE, FAAN, ANEF; and Karen West, MSN RN; of my colleagues from the American Nursing Informatics Association, including Cheryl D. Parker PhD, MSN, RN-BC, CNE, FHIMSS; and to my technological wizard and husband, James Sipes, BEE, MSEE.

Janet Weber, EdD, RN, had the idea for this book as part of a series on basic topics nurses need to know to practice today. She also provided constructive criticism to ensure this volume met the series' guidelines, including the case scenarios, critical thinking activities, and study questions.

PART I

FOUNDATIONS OF NURSING INFORMATICS

CHAPTER 1

NURSING INFORMATICS: DEFINITION, EVOLUTION, GUIDING PRINCIPLES, EXPECTATIONS

CAROLYN SIPES

LEARNING OBJECTIVES AND OUTCOMES

Upon completion of this chapter, the reader will be able to:

- Define nursing informatics (NI), health informatics, and consumer health informatics.
- List three driving forces that influenced the development of a skilled workforce for 2020 and beyond.
- Discuss why nurses need to develop NI skills.
- List two basic guiding principles of NI that all nurses need to know.
- List two American Association of Colleges of Nursing (AACN) Essentials related to NI and discuss why they are important.
- List three Quality and Safety Education for Nurses (QSEN) competencies related to NI.
- Discuss areas in clinical practice where he or she will apply NI.

☉ KEY NURSING INFORMATICS TERMS AND ORGANIZATIONS

Some of the key concepts and terms you will hear in the discipline of nursing informatics (NI) are included here. The professional organizations listed provide the guidelines and standards for NI practice.

⊙ KEY NURSING INFORMATICS TERMS (*continued*)

American Association of Colleges of Nursing (AACN)

American Medical Informatics Association (AMIA)

American Nurses Association (ANA)

American Nursing Informatics Association (ANIA)

Computer literacy

Consumer health informatics

Electronic health record (EHR)

Electronic medical record (EMR)

Health informatics

Informatics

Information technology (IT)

Institute of Medicine (IOM)

National League for Nursing (NLN)

Nursing informatics (NI)

Quality and Safety Education for Nurses Institute (QSEN)

Technology

World Health Organization (WHO)

INTRODUCTION: THE DISCIPLINE OF NURSING INFORMATICS

What are some of your experiences with informatics at work and in your associate degree program? Have you been involved in an EHR implementation during which you used technology to document patient information?

Consider some of the general experiences you have in your current practice environment. Do you use informatics to document in your job role? What is your definition of NI?

What you already know from your practice and what you have learned from an associate degree program will provide the answers to these questions, especially if you have been involved with an EHR implementation through which you began to develop informatics skills and an understanding of what informatics is. These considerations may also stimulate curiosity regarding how informatics skills can be developed if you have not had the opportunities to do so yet.

■ Questions to Consider Before Reading On

1. *What are the differences among NI, health informatics, and consumer health informatics?*

2. *Did you know nursing informatics is a discipline unto itself? What do you think this might include?*

3. *How do you think understanding the discipline of nursing informatics might apply to your practice? What are some of the skills taken from NI that you might use?*

What Is Nursing Informatics?

Nursing Informatics, as a new, evolving discipline, is an established specialty within nursing. Its definition is the fundamental element shaping the specialty. The definition guides role description for nurses interested in informatics and recommends components of practice, education, training, and research, and supports the legitimacy of the practice and the general competencies of a nurse who specializes in informatics. The definition is the introductory element shaping documents of national scope for the NI specialty. In addition, the definition is used by funding agencies to outline projects and fund NI efforts, such as the Division of Nursing in the Department of Health and Human Services (DHHS) and the National Institute for Nursing Research (NINR).

The profession of nursing was among the first health disciplines to embrace informatics through its recognition of NI as a specialty practice area (Bickford, 2015). In little over two decades, NI has evolved into an expanding body of knowledge, confirming and supporting its relevance and applicability to all domains of nursing (e.g., education, research, practice, information management and technology, administration).

The evolution of NI is apparent in the establishment of many higher educational NI programs. Its growth is seen through the development of professional organizations dedicated to NI, as standards and scope of practice are set, and certification is made possible (Anderson & Sensmeier, 2014; Bickford, 2015; HIMSS Nursing Informatics Awareness Task Force, 2007). The Technology Informatics Guiding Education Reform (TIGER; n.d.) project in the United States (Fung, 2016; Schlak & Troseth, 2013; Staggers, Gassert, & Curran, 2001, 2002) has facilitated and promoted NI in practice and in academia to improve and support better overall quality of care for patients.

The TIGER initiative began in 2006 as the result of nursing leaders coming together to harness the benefits of EHRs for the nursing profession (Hebda & Czar, 2013). The goals of the TIGER summit were to improve patient care through use of informatics and technology by the healthcare team. The work of the TIGER initiative has produced measurable results in competency implementation and validation (ANA, 2015a). Currently, 21 countries have come together through this initiative TIGER to create international informatics competencies that incorporate evidence-based research and technology that will improve patient care globally. Today, the TIGER initiative is responsible for developing what is known as the *Health Information Technology Competencies (HITCOMP)* tool, which is used to assess informatics competences on a universal scale.

Informatics Definitions

There are a number of different definitions of informatics; the three listed here are the ones most frequently used. The ANA (2015a) defined *NI* as "the specialty that integrates nursing science with multiple information and analytical sciences to identify, define, manage, and communicate data, information, knowledge, and wisdom in nursing practice (pp. 1–2)". Examples of how these might be used are discussed in the following text. NI supports nurses, consumers, patients, the interprofessional healthcare team, and other stakeholders in their decision-making in all roles and settings to achieve desired outcomes. This support is accomplished through the use of information structures, information processes, and information technology (IT).

The AMIA defines *consumer health informatics* as "the field devoted to informatics from multiple consumer or patient views. These include patient-focused informatics, health literacy and consumer education" (p. 1). The focus of this type of informatics is different; it emphasizes "information structures and processes that empower consumers to manage their own health—for example health information literacy, consumer-friendly language, personal health records, and Internet-based strategies and resources" (AMIA, 2018, p. 1). *Health informatics*, defined by the U.S. National Library of Medicine, is "the interdisciplinary study of the design, development, adoption, and application of IT-based innovations in healthcare services delivery, management, and planning (p. 1)."

The ANA includes the advancement of outcomes for population heath in their informatics framework (ANA, 2015b, p. 2). When nurses have a degree of informatics proficiency, they are better equipped to manage patients' complex medical data and provide high-quality patient care as well as support consumers, the interprofessional healthcare team, and other stakeholders in their decision-making in all roles and settings to achieve desired outcomes. Nurse informaticists work to advance healthcare as developers of communication and information technologies, researchers, chief nursing officers (CNOs), chief information officers (CIOs), software engineers, implementation consultants, and policy developers. This support is accomplished through the use of information structures, information processes, and IT.

Other definitions vary, but, in general, NI is an integration of computer and nursing science to convey "data information, knowledge, and wisdom in nursing practice" (ANA, 2015b, p. 2). Because the use of technology is extensive, every aspect of nursing practice falls within the category of an informatics nurse (IN), regardless of whether she or he has board certification or not (ANA, 2015b).

▓ Questions to Consider Before Reading On

1. *How do professional organizations influence, identify needs, and push for NI competencies and skills development?*

2. *Why do nurses need to develop NI skills and knowledge? What are some ways the knowledge of NI will support you in your practice?*

3. *How would you assess your current knowledge and skills level regarding NI?*

▓ Driving Forces and the Evolution of Nursing Informatics

Many professional organizations realized early on that the integration of computers and other high-tech processes into the practice of healthcare would change how that care is provided today. These organizations provided the first recommendations intended to meet the needs of the high-tech nursing workforce of the future, when they realized they needed to provide improved quality and safety of patient care today, especially through the use of computer technology.

Examples of the competencies they identified include computer skills and literacy, informatics knowledge and ability used to organize and collect data to improve practice by all nurses for the sake of patient safety and outcomes of care.

Historically, the IOM (2003) identified five core competencies needed by all health-care care providers. Two of the five specifically define informatics requirements:

- Focus on quality improvement (QI) and
- Apply informatics skills and competencies—where informatics is defined as: Communication, managing knowledge, mitigating error, and supporting decision-making through use of IT.

In 2008, both the American Association of Colleges of Nursing (AACN) and the National League of Nursing (NLN) emphasized that knowledge and skills in information management and patient care technology (informatics) are critical components in nursing education and accreditation. At this time, many also identified that informatics competencies and skills were seriously lacking in nursing education and practice.

The IOM prepared a groundbreaking report, *The Future of Nursing: Leading Change, Advancing Health* (2010), which looked 10 years to the future of nursing practice and suggested that the nursing workforce of 2020 will primarily be technology based, requiring high-tech informatics skills. This report was driven by the legislation of the Affordable Care Act (ACA, 2010) and its objective to overhaul the healthcare system.

The NLN (2015) issued a recent call for further action to prepare students for a technological (informatics) future in healthcare, highlighting a clear need for nursing education "to teach with and about technology (informatics) to better inform healthcare interventions that improve healthcare outcomes and prepare the nursing workforce" (p. 4).

You will see the terms informatics nurse (IN) used interchangeably with the term nurse informatisists (NI), depending on their organization's definitions. Both are used in ANA's (2015b) *Nursing Informatics: Scope and Standards of Practice* Both terms, *informatics nurse* and *nurse informaticist*, refer to the nurse who has basic informatics skills, knowledge, and competencies as compared to the informatics nurse specialist (INS), who has at minimum a master's degree and advanced expertise.

CASE SCENARIO

Jill has been working in a healthcare facility that is still using a paper-based system in which she documents patient information into a paper medical record every day. She has just found out that her facility will start implementing an electronic health system (EHR) system in the next 6 months. She has been told that she will need to start working to develop informatics skills so that she will become more competent when documenting patient information. She is reluctant to do this because the way she has been documenting patient information over

(continued)

(continued)

the past 10 years is satisfactory and she feels she does not need to learn to use the new electronic medical record (EMR) system.
Questions Jill begins to consider:

1. What are some of the benefits of a new EHR?
2. Will there be training and support available to teach me the new system?
3. If training is available, how long will it take?

■ Questions to Consider Before Reading On

What would you need to do in order to better understand the value and benefits of the new EHR?

You begin to evaluate and discuss the skills you will need to use the new EHR system and ask questions such as:

1. *What are the first basic skills I need to develop to be able to document my patient's information in the new system?*

■ Why Do Nurses Need to Develop Nursing Informatics Skills?

The IOM (2010) report reviewed how nurses' roles, responsibilities, and educational needs must change to meet the needs of an aging, increasingly diverse population and indicated that the should respond to the more complex, technology-rich healthcare system with the increased use of informatics. One of the key recommendations to come out of the report is the recommendation that by 2020, 80% of practicing nurses should have more education in NI and should achieve an advanced degree, defined as a bachelor of science in nursing (BSN).

Based on *The Future of Nursing: Leading Change, Advancing Health* (IOM, 2010) and focused on transforming the nursing profession, the IOM report was used as a framework to recommend skills and education needed by all nurses in the new high-tech healthcare environment. Today, patient healthcare needs and care have become more complex, yet often nurses' knowledge, skills, and competencies have not kept up with the changes required to provide safe, high-quality, high-tech healthcare.

Certain basic competencies suggested include the need for nurses to use technology to:

■ Collect evidence-based research to improve practice.

■ Develop information, computer literacy, and skills in order to effectively use an EMR and other clinical systems.

■ Create healthcare polices through data collection.

■ Develop specific competencies related to the areas of practice such as

○ Use of telehealth in community health.

○ Use of medical devices in all clinical practice areas.

■ With high-tech nursing practice and use of EHRs, nurses with computer skills and understanding of informatics are needed to facilitate communication with other interdisciplinary teams as well as with IT.

To achieve an understanding of the informatics skills, knowledge, and competencies required in today's high-tech healthcare environments, the IOM (2010) urged that nurses achieve higher levels of education and educators use newer methods and technology. Further, the report noted that other areas where informatics competencies are needed include workforce planning and policy making based on data collection, both of which require use of technology and computer skills, an essential component of nursing education.

The World Health Organization (WHO) also has a number of informatics initiatives in place to help meet its e-Health mandate, which includes the eHealth Technical Advisory Group formed solely to support WHO's work in e-Health (WHO, 2015); the WHO is another organization that recognizes the need for nurses to possess informatics competencies and skills. The NLN (2015) also identified the need to prepare students for technological/digital healthcare through the nursing education "to teach … about technology (informatics) to better inform healthcare interventions that improve healthcare outcomes and prepare the nursing workforce" (p. 4).

As mentioned, professional organizations recognized the need for and recommended specific competencies all nurses must have in today's high-tech healthcare environment. Other such competencies are discussed later in this chapter. The Quality and Safety Education for Nurses (QSEN) Institute initiative that specifically defines knowledge, skills, and attitudes (KSAs) related to NI is discussed in Box 1.3.

■ Questions to Consider Before Reading On

1. *What are two reasons nurses need to have NI and technology skills?*
2. *Which organizations developed guidelines and standards of practice for nursing informaticists?*
3. *Why is it important to understand the NI guidelines? How do they apply to your practice?*

■ Guiding Principles of Nursing Informatics Practice

With the rapid evolution of NI, many organizations are beginning to recognize the impact and value NI professionals can have on the quality of patient care, including improved safety. Nurse informaticists impact workflow, facilitate communication between IT and nursing, as well as support more acceptance of clinical systems used in healthcare on a daily basis (Health, Information and Management Systems Society [HIMSS], 2014).

A number of organizations have provided guidelines and standards of practice for the discipline of NI. Of these, there are the ANA's (2015b) *Nursing Informatics: Scope and Standards of Practice*, AACN, Commission on Collegiate Nursing Education (CCNE), the QSEN initiative supported by the Robert Wood Johnson Foundation (RWJF), and the TIGER initiative, to name a few.

Regardless of the organizational framework used or regulatory body, all organizations and regulatory agencies are in consensus that there is a need for all nurses to understand these basic guiding principles and have NI knowledge, skills, and competencies in order to practice better, high-quality, safer patient care. The contributions of the different organizations are discussed in the following text.

American Nurses Association

The ANA has developed its own standards and scope of practice for NI. *Nursing Informatics: The Scope and Standards of Practice* (ANA, 2015b) describe the common performance, level of care, and quality of practice for which nurses are accountable. There are two main levels of standards for NI—the NI standards of practice and the professional performance standards.

The Standards of Practice for Nursing Informatics are guidelines for practice that have both general and specific recommendations for the specialty; general recommendations follow the nursing process of assessment, planning, outcome planning, diagnosis, implementation, and evaluation. Standards of Professional Performance for Nursing Informatics speak to the nursing role with regard to ethics, research, education, and resource utilization.

An overview of the ANA's (2015b) *Nursing Informatics: Scope and Standards of Practice* is presented in Box 1.1, which includes the six Standards of Practice and 10 Standards of Professional Performance for Nursing Informatics as defined by the ANA (2015).

BOX 1.1

ANA's *NURSING INFORMATICS: SCOPE AND STANDARDS OF PRACTICE*

STANDARDS OF PRACTICE FOR NURSING INFORMATICS	STANDARDS OF PROFESSIONAL PERFORMANCE FOR NURSING INFORMATICS
Assessment	Ethics
Diagnosis, problems, and issues identification	Education
Outcomes identification	Evidence-based practice and research
Planning	Quality of practice
Implementation	Communication
Evaluation	Leadership

(continued)

BOX 1.1 *(continued)*

STANDARDS OF PRACTICE FOR NURSING INFORMATICS	STANDARDS OF PROFESSIONAL PERFORMANCE FOR NURSING INFORMATICS
	Collaboration
	Profession practice evaluation Resource utilization Environmental health

ANA, American Nurses Association.

SOURCE: American Nurses Association. (2015b). *Nursing informatics: Scope and standards of practice* (pp. 68–94). Silver Spring, MD: Author.

American Association of Colleges of Nursing

In 2006, the AACN convened a taskforce which identified competencies including those for informatics, which should be achieved by professional nurses to achieve high-quality and safe patient care (Box 1.2). An overview of the major competencies were identified in the following areas:

- Critical thinking
- Healthcare systems and policies
- Communication
- Illness and disease management
- Ethics
- Information and healthcare technologies

The AACN Essentials needed by nurses that specifically apply to nursing informatics competencies, skills, and knowledge include Essential IV listed in Box 1.2.

BOX 1.2

AACN ESSENTIALS

SELECTED NURSING INFORMATICS ESSENTIALS APPLICABLE TO INFORMATICS	
Essential II	Basic Organizational and Systems Leadership for Quality Care and Patient Safety
Essential III	Scholarship for Evidence-Based Practice
Essential IV	Information Management and Application of Patient Care Technology

(continued)

BOX 1.2 (*continued*)

SELECTED NURSING INFORMATICS ESSENTIALS APPLICABLE TO INFORMATICS	
Essential V	Healthcare Policy, Finance, and Regulatory Environments
Essential VI	Interprofessional Communication and Collaboration for Improving Patient Health Outcomes
Essential IX	Baccalaureate Generalist Nursing Practice

AACN, American Association of Colleges of Nursing.

SOURCE: American Association of Colleges of Nursing (2008). AACN essentials; Baccalaureate essentials. Retrieved from https://www.aacnnursing.org/Education-Resources/AACN-Essentials.

The AACN (2008) further defined specific skills needed by the baccalaureate graduate, which are different from the Essentials needed in master of science in nursing and doctor of nursing practice graduate programs:

1. Demonstrate skills in using patient care technologies, information systems, and communication devices that support safe nursing practice.

2. Use telecommunication technologies to assist in effective communication in a variety of healthcare settings.

3. Apply safeguards and decision-making support tools embedded in patient care technologies and information systems to support a safe practice environment for both patients and healthcare workers.

4. Understand the use of computer information systems (CIS) to document interventions related to achieving nurse-sensitive outcomes.

5. Use standardized terminology in a care environment that reflects nursing's unique contribution to patient outcomes.

6. Evaluate data from all relevant sources, including technology, to inform the delivery of care.

7. Recognize the role of IT in improving patient care outcomes and creating a safe care environment.

8. Uphold ethical standards related to data security, regulatory requirements, confidentiality, and clients' right to privacy.

9. Apply patient care technologies as appropriate to address the needs of a diverse patient population.

10. Advocate for the use of new patient care technologies for safe, quality care.

11. Recognize that redesign of workflow and care processes should precede implementation of care technology to facilitate nursing practice.

12. Participate in evaluation of information systems in practice settings through policy and procedure development (AACN Baccalaureate Education, 2008).

Each of the Essentials listed above will be discussed in the chapter relevant to chapter content.

Commission on Collegiate Nursing Education

The CCNE, which falls under the umbrella of the AACN, ensures nursing programs meet a certain set of quality standards. The scope of CCNE includes the accreditation of BSN and NI degree programs. Its purpose is to accredit BSN programs that are in compliance with standards of practice as defined and required by other organizations and to monitor programs' continuous quality-improvement (CQI) efforts. The CCNE recognizes that education plays a key role in nurses being able to build the fundamental knowledge, skills, and competencies necessary to become leaders as well as public advocates for their patients and profession (CCNE, 2017).

Quality and Safety Education for Nurses

The overall goal of the QSEN initiative is to meet the challenge of preparing future nurses who will have the knowledge, skills and attitudes (KSAs) necessary to provide high quality safe healthcare (Cronenwett et al., 2007). Gaps were identified in NI knowledge, education, and skills required for nurses to competently use EHRs to provide patient care (Cronenwett et al., 2007; Disch, Barnsteiner, & McGuinn, 2013). This initiative is discussed in subsequent chapters as it applies to their specific content.

Based on the IOM recommendations, the QSEN initiative developed NI competencies that closely examine the nursing KSAs needed in BSN programs. Of the six key areas involved in KSA competencies, the most relevant here include quailty improvement, patient safety, and informatics (Bryant, Whitehead, & Kleier, 2016; Guillermo, & Orta, 2016).

The KSA definitions for NI as well as sets of KSAs for the informatics competencies that were created for use in nursing prelicensure programs and BSN education programs are listed in Box 1.3. These are suggested as guides for NI curricular development, and allow transition to practice or to other education programs. You will see QSEN KSAs in other chapters as they are integrated into various topics.

BOX 1.3

QUALITY AND SAFETY EDUCATION FOR NURSES

QSEN: KSAs TO PREPARE FUTURE NURSES

Informatics defined: Informatics is the use of information and technology to communicate, manage knowledge, mitigate error, and support decision-making (QSEN, 2007).

Explain why information and technology skills are essential for safe patient care (knowledge).

Seek education about how information is managed in care settings before providing care (skills).

Appreciate the need for all health professionals to seek lifelong, continuous learning of information technology skills (attitudes).

(continued)

BOX 1.3 (*continued*)

QSEN: KSAs TO PREPARE FUTURE NURSES

Identify essential information that must be available in a common database to support patient care; contrast benefits and limitations of different communication technologies and their impact on safety and quality (knowledge).

Navigate the EHR; document and plan patient care in an EHR; employ communication technologies to coordinate care for patients (skills).

Value technologies that support clinical decision-making, error prevention, and care coordination.

Protect confidentiality of health information in EHRs (attitudes).

Describe examples of how technology and information management are related to the quality and safety of patient care; recognize the time, effort, and skill required for computers, databases, and other technologies to become reliable and effective tools for patient care (knowledge).

Respond appropriately to clinical decision-making supports and alerts; use information-management tools to monitor outcomes of care processes; use high-quality electronic sources of healthcare information (skills).

Value nurses' involvement in design, selection, implementation, and evaluation of information technologies to support patient care (attitudes).

KSA, knowledge, skills, attitudes; QSEN, Quality and Safety Education for Nurses.

SOURCE: Adapted from Cronenwett, L., Sherwood, G., Barnsteiner, J., Disch, J., Johnson, J., Mitchell, P., . . . Warren, J. (2007). Quality and safety education for nurses. *Nursing Outlook, 55*(3), 122–131. doi:10.1016/j.outlook.2007.02.006

QSEN SCENARIO

You have been asked to explain why information and technology (nursing informatics) skills are essential for the practice of safe patient care. How would you respond?

▒ Questions to Consider Before Reading On

1. *What is the difference between the nurse informaticist and the INS?*

2. *Discuss two standards of practice for the nurse informaticist. List how to apply competency examples to the standards of practice.*

3. *What challenges and opportunities await the nurses of 2025?*

▨ Professional Nurse Expectations: Application of Nursing Informatics to Practice

As discussed previously, NI is the specialty that integrates nursing science with multiple information and analytical sciences to identify, define, manage, and communicate data, information, knowledge, and wisdom in nursing practice. For many, NI and healthcare informatics are about technology. Queries raised by recent researchers pose the questions—as technology becomes more ubiquitous, is there a need to focus on computer literacy, knowledge, and skills (Skiba, 2017)? Should the focus be on digital literacy? This is particularly true if EHRs are required of all care facilities. Many of these questions will be explored in future chapters of this textbook.

Risling (2017) suggested that the pace of technological evolution in healthcare is advancing as discussed previously. Key technological trends that are likely to influence nursing practice and education over the next decade have been discussed by many professional organizations. The complexity of curricular revision will create challenges due to rapid practice change. Nurse educators are encouraged to consider the role of EHRs, wearable technologies, big data and data analytics, and increased patient engagement as key areas for curriculum development. Student nurses, and those already in practice, should be offered ongoing educational opportunities to enhance a wide spectrum of professional informatics skills. A key consideration is that the nurses of 2025 will most certainly inhabit a very different practice environment than the one that exists today and technology will be key in this transformation (Risling, 2017).

The ANA's 16 NI standards, which provide a framework for evaluating practice outcomes and goals, are those to which all informatics nurses are held accountable in practice. The set of specific NI competencies accompanying each standard serves as essential evidence of compliance with that standard (ANA, 2015b). The six Standards of Practice for Nursing Informatics are defined in Box 1.4 and include activities demonstrating competency requirements for RNs in their practice area. The ANA textbook, *Nursing Informatics: Scope and Standards of Practice*, includes details of the many competencies that meet these standards (ANA, 2015b, pp. 68–94). Box 1.5 explores the 10 professional performance competency standards for the nurse informaticist (Box 1.5).

The standards identified and the competency examples provided in Boxes 1.4 and 1.5 are the expected, basic NI levels required for BSN nurses. ANA's *Nursing Informatics: Scope and Standards of Practice* (2015b) also lists competencies expected at the advanced NI level, the INS, for those with an MSN degree. Additional competencies expected of the INS are listed within the same basic standards used for the NI.

BOX 1.4

STANDARDS OF PRACTICE FOR NURSING INFORMATICS

Standard 1: Assessment	The NI collects comprehensive data, information, and emerging evidence pertinent to the situation. Competency example: Uses workflow analysis to examine current practice, workflow, and the potential impact of an informatics solution on that workflow.
Standard 2: Diagnosis, problems, and issues identification	The NI analyzes assessment data to identify diagnoses, problems, issues, and opportunities for improvement. Competency example: Validates the diagnoses, problems, needs, issues, and opportunities for improvement with the healthcare consumer—this links standards 1 and 2.
Standard 3: Outcomes identification	The NI identifies expected outcomes for a plan individualized to the healthcare consumer. Competency example: Documents expected outcome as measurable goals.
Standard 4: Planning	The NI develops a plan that prescribes strategies, alternatives, and recommendations to attain expected outcomes. Competency example: Develops the plan in collaboration with the healthcare consumer and key stakeholders.
Standard 5: Implementation	The NI implements the plan. Competency example: Uses specific evidence-based actions and processes to resolve diagnoses, problems, or issues to achieve outcomes. The informatics nurse (a) coordinates planned activities, (b) employs informatics solutions, and (c) provides consultation to influence the identified plan.
Standard 6: Evaluation	The NI evaluates progress toward attainment of outcomes. Competency example: Conducts a systematic evaluation of outcomes.

NI, nurse informaticist.

BOX 1.5

STANDARDS OF PROFESSIONAL PERFORMANCE FOR NURSING INFORMATICS

Standard 7: Ethics	The NI practices ethically: Competency example: Applies the *Code of Ethics for Nurses with Interpretative Statements* to guide practice (ANA, 2001).
Standard 8: Education	The NI addresses the need to education, attains knowledge and competence reflecting current nursing practice. Competency example: Demonstrates commitment to lifelong learning.

(continued)

BOX 1.5 (*continued*)

Standard 9 Evidence-based practice and research	The NI integrates evidence and research into practice. Competency example: Demonstrates application and integration of evidence and research into practice.
Standard 10: Quality of practice	The NI contributes to the quality and effectiveness of nursing and informatics practice. Competency example: Collects data to analyze and monitor quality of informatics practice.
Standard 11: Communication	The NI communicates effectively. Competency example: Communicates effectively using a variety of methods.
Standard 12: Leadership	The NI demonstrates leadership in professional practice. Competency example: Demonstrates leadership skills. such as mentoring and problem solving, and promotes the organization's mission and vision.
Standard 13: Collaboration	The NI collaborates with the healthcare consumer and others in the practice of nursing and nursing informatics. Competency example: Partners with others to effect change—this links standards 12 and 13.
Standard 14: Professional practice evaluation	The NI evaluates her or his own nursing and informatics practice. Competency example: Self-evaluations identify areas of strength as well as areas for professional growth.
Standard 15: Resource utilization	The NI uses appropriate resources to plan and implement safe practices. Competency example: Modifies practice as discipline and technology evolves.
Standard 16: Environmental health	The NI supports nursing practice in a safe and healthy environment. Competency example: Participates in ways to support healthy communities.

Critical Thinking Questions and Activities

- *As you review the skills, knowledge, and competencies listed above for the MSN and DNP graduates, how do these apply to what you currently know and practice?*

- *Explain how you might apply each of the professional practice competency examples identified in standards 2 and 3 provided in Box 1.4. What are some examples found in your practice?*

- *Explain how you would meet professional performance standards 10 and 13 described in Box 1.5. What are some examples in your practice?*

- *Explore the QSEN KSAs discussed earlier. Select one of the KSAs and discuss how you would apply that to your practice.*

SUMMARY

The definition, history, and evolution of NI were discussed as were many of the driving forces used to evaluate then provide recommendations to meet the needs of the 2020 and 2030 workforce today.

The reason nurses need to develop informatics skills, based on a number of reports, including the very influential IOM (2010) report, was described. To meet this growing need for new skill, the IOM (2010) urged nurses to achieve higher levels of education; the need for education in NI as well as lists of competencies offered by many national nursing organizations were described. The profession of nursing was among the first health disciplines to embrace informatics through the recognition of NI as a specialty practice area.

A number of organizations have provided guidelines for the practice and discipline of NI. Of these, there are the ANA Standards and Scope of Practice for Nursing Informatics, AACN, and CCNE, the QSEN initiative supported by RWJF, and the TIGER initiative. Each of these organizations developed standards and competencies required to function at the basic NI level and are provided in detail and include examples of application to practice as the NI.

■ References

Affordable Care Act (ACA). (2010). Retrieved from https://www.healthinsurance.org/glossary/affordable-care-act/September, 2018.

American Association of Colleges of Nursing (2008). AACN essentials; Baccalaureate essentials. Retrieved from https://www.aacnnursing.org/Education-Resources/AACN-Essentials.

American Medical Informatics Association (AMIA). (2018). Consumer health informatics, Retrieved from https://www.amia.org/applications-informatics/consumer-health-informatics. October.

American Nurses Association. (2015a). Health IT initiatives. Retrieved from http://nursingworld.org/MainMenuCaterfories/The Practice of Professional Nursing/Health-IT.org

American Nurses Association. (2015b). *Nursing informatics: Scope and standards of practice* (pp. 68–94). Silver Spring, MD: Author.

Anderson, C., & Sensmeier, J. (2014). Nursing informatics: A specialty on the rise. *Nursing Management, 45*(6), 16–18. doi:10.1097/01.NUMA.0000449768.37489.ac

Bickford, C. J. (2015). The specialty of nursing informatics: New scope and standards guide practice. *CIN: Computers, Informatics, Nursing, 33*(4), 129–131. doi:10.1097/CIN.0000000000000150

Bryant, L., Whitehead, D., & Kleier, J. (2016). Development and testing of an instrument to measure informatics knowledge, skills, and attitudes among entry-level nursing students. *Online Journal of Nursing Informatics, 20*(2). Retrieved from http://www.himss.org/ojni

Commission on Collegiate Nursing Education. (2017). Procedures for accreditation of baccalaureate and graduate degree nursing programs. Retrieved from https://www.aacnnursing.org/Portals/42/CCNE/PDF/Procedures.pdf

Cronenwett, L., Sherwood, G., Barnsteiner, J., Disch, J., Johnson, J., Mitchell, P., ... Warren, J. (2007). Quality and safety education for nurses. *Nursing Outlook, 55*(3), 122–131. doi:10.1016/j.outlook.2007.02.006

Disch, J., Barnsteiner, J., & McGuinn, K. (2013). Taking a "deep dive" on integrating QSEN content in San Francisco Bay Area schools of nursing. *Journal of Professional Nursing, 29*(2), 75–81. doi:10.1016/j.profnurs.2012.12.007

Fung, K. Y. M. (2016). Utilizing TIGER competencies to improve informatics practice. *Doctor of Nursing Practice (DNP) Projects, 76.* Retrieved from https://repository.usfca.edu/dnp/76

Guillermo, V., & Orta, R. (2016, March 21). *Making the most out of QSEN's Knowledge, Attitude and Skills (KAS) competencies in an RN to BSN program: A three level education approach.* 43rd Biennial Convention, Sigma Theta Tau International, Las Vegas, NV.

Healthcare Information and Management Systems Society (HIMSS). (2007). An emerging giant: Nursing informatics. Retreived from https://www.himss.org/emerging-giant-nursing -informatics.

Healthcare Information and Management Systems Society. (2014). Health informatics defined. Retrieved from https://www.himss.org/health-informatics-defined

Hebda, T. & Czar , P. (2013). *Handbook of informatics for nurses and healthcare professionals* (5th ed.). New York, NY: Pearson.

Institute of Medicine. (2003). *Health professions education: A bridge to quality.* Washington, DC: National Academies Press.

Institute of Medicine. (2004). *Keeping patients safe: Transforming the work environment of nurses.* Washington, DC: National Academies Press.

Institute of Medicine. (2010). *The future of nursing: Leading change, advancing health.* Washington, DC: National Academies Press. Retrieved from http://wwwthefutureofnursing.org

National League for Nursing. (2015). *A VISION for the changing faculty role: Preparing students for the technological world of health care.* Washington, DC: Author.

Risling, T. (2017). Educating the nurses of 2025: Technology trends of the next decade. *Nurse Education in Practice, 22,* 89–92. doi:10.1016/j.nepr.2016.12.007

Schlak, S. E., & Troseth, M. (2013). TIGER initiative: Advancing health IT. *Nursing Management, 44*(1), 19–20. doi:10.1097/01.NUMA.0000424025.21411.be

Skiba, D. (2017). Nursing informatics education: From automation to connected care. In J. Murphy, W. Goossen, & P. Weber (Eds.), *Forecasting informatics competencies for nurses in the future of connected health* (pp. 9–19). Amsterdam, the Netherlands: IMIA and IOS Press.

Staggers, N., Gassert, C. A., & Curran, C. (2001). Informatics competencies for nurses at four levels of practice. *Journal of Nursing Education, 40*(7), 303–316. Retrieved from https:// www.learntechlib.org/p/93916/

Staggers, N., Gassert, C. A., & Curran, C. (2002). A Delphi study to determine informatics competencies for nurses at four levels of practice. *Nursing Research, 51*(6), 383–390. doi:10.1097/00006199-200211000-00006

Technology Informatics Guiding education reform. (n.d.). Informatics competencies for every registered nurse: Recommendations from the TIGER collaborative. Retrieved from https://www.himss.org/professionaldevelopment/tiger-initiative

World Health Organization. (2015). eHealth collaborations. Retrieved from http://www.who .int/ehealth/about/ehealthcollaborations/en

CHAPTER 2

NURSING INFORMATICS: ROLES, PROFESSIONAL ORGANIZATIONS, AND THEORIES

CAROLYN SIPES

LEARNING OBJECTIVES AND OUTCOMES

Upon completion of this chapter, the reader will be able to:

- Discuss three nursing informatics roles. How are these different from other nursing roles?
- Discuss three nursing informatics organizations.
- List three levels of Benner's Novice-to-Expert Model.
- What does *DIKW* mean? How can it be applied to your practice?
- Describe two theories and how they support the discipline of nursing informatics.

⊙ KEY NURSING INFORMATICS TERMS

Some of the key concepts, terms, and organizations you will hear in the discipline of nursing informatics are:

American Nursing Informatics Association (ANIA)

American Health Information Management Association (AHIMA)

Alliance for Nursing Informatics (ANI)

Benner's Novice-to-Expert Model

Competencies

Chaos Theory

Change Theory

Cognitive Science

Computer Science

Data–information–knowledge–wisdom (DIKW)

Healthcare Information and Management Systems Society (HIMSS)

⊙ KEY NURSING INFORMATICS TERMS (*continued*)

International Medical Informatics Association (IMIA)

Informatics

Knowledge

Sigma Theta Tau International (STTI)

Wisdom

INTRODUCTION: NURSING INFORMATICS ROLES AND ORGANIZATIONS

This chapter provides an overview of roles you might expect to see and experience in nursing informatics (NI). You will find selected key organizations that both support informatics and are specific to NI. It also provides background of some of the nursing theories and explains how they might relate to the specialty of NI.

Consider what you already know regarding the roles of a nurse informaticist (NI) and the different informatics organizations that support role development. Based on this, what do you think is needed in the way of further education regarding skills, knowledge, and competency in today's nursing workforce?

What have your experiences been with informatics at work and in your associate degree program? Have you been involved in an electronic health record (EHR) implementation in which you learned to use technology to document patient information? Consider some of the general experiences you have in your current practice environment. How do you understand and define *informatics*?

As you reflect on each of these questions, you may realize you already have considerable experience and knowledge regarding the value of professional organizations, such as providing continuing-education programs for skill development or education related to a new trend in patient care.

▨ Questions to Consider Before Reading On

1. *What is the difference between competency and skill?*
2. *What role might the bachelor of science in nursing (BSN) informatics nurse (IN) assume with the implementation of an EHR? How does knowing this help you to understand more about the IN role and how it applies to all nurses?*
3. *Discuss two basic competencies and skills needed by a BSN in practice. Are these the same you might see and use in NI?*
4. *What do you currently understand about how nursing theories support NI?*

▨ Roles of Nurse Informaticists

According to the *Nursing Informatics Scope and Standards of Practice*, those who enter the NI field because of an interest or experience in informatics are INs, also known as NI depending on the organization. A nurse with either a graduate education degree in NI or field experiences related to informatics as the advanced MSN degree is an informatics nurse specialist (INS; American Nurses Association [ANA], 2015b, p. 17). The roles of INs vary with the job and their specialty in healthcare, but the general focus of NI is on seven areas originally defined by the National Institutes of Health, National Center for Nursing Research (NCNR) Priority Expert Panel on NI (Pillar & Golumbic, 1993). The roles have evolved greatly since then, but the seven basic skills are foundational to many organizations.

The initial seven IN roles were (Pillar & Golumbic, 1993):

- Using data, information, and knowledge applied to patient care
- Defining data in patient care
- Acquiring and delivering patient care knowledge
- Creating new tools for patient care from new technologies
- Applying ergonomics to nurse–computer interfaces
- Integrating systems
- Evaluating the effects of nursing systems

These were defined in terms generic enough that they still apply today. Roles are inclusive of competencies and skills as well as knowledge but what is the difference between the roles?

Skills Versus Competencies

The major difference between skills and competencies is one of scope: competencies define the requirements for success on the job in broader, more inclusive terms than skills do. Think of skills as one of three aspects that make up a competency: the other two are knowledge and abilities.

Today the IN or even those with NI experience from on-the-job training and skills gained in a wide variety of roles, especially with the evolution of healthcare to a high-tech industry. Nurses working in informatics today are functioning at increased levels of complexity, and expectations for enterprise systems are great. With this said, it is important to understand that there is great deal of overlap in job roles and job descriptions. Understanding basic role expectations and functions is key, as is the INs work with other clinical nurses to improve clinical systems.

Nurse informatics interact with a variety of healthcare professionals at many organizational levels, from the clinical nurse to the chief executive officer; therefore, opportunities for collaboration in decision-making are critical. Some of the basic informatics competencies once accredited to informatics specialists have only now become mandatory for all nurses, including clinical, educational, and administrative roles (ANA, 2015). Further, the basic level of competencies and skills needed to participate in the development and implementation of an electronic medical record/EHR has become much more complex. (The term *EHR* is more inclusive and accepted today as it includes more than just the hospital record, but you may still see the term *EMR* used.) Overall, the scope and practice of all NI—basic to advanced—will continue to expand with the advancement of high-tech innovations as they are applied to the healthcare industry.

To be specific, some of the roles now expected of the IN include those listed here, but as noted earlier, this list is not inclusive as the NI discipline continues to evolve as expectations and knowledge flourish and expand.

With implementation of an EHR and EMR, expectations include:

- Ability to conduct workflow analyses
- Ability to prioritize data-collection activities in order to analyze data for reports
- Use of analytical models, algorithms, and other tools for assessment and evaluation
- Ability to differentiate and apply tools to collect outcomes information, participate in planning, and contribute on teams during the design, implementation, and evaluation of information systems

In clinical practice, NI skills and roles involve the use of devices and hardware—as all nurses use devices—that are summarized here but discussed in more detail in later chapters.

New integrated technologies evolve every day. Some of these include:

- The use of smartphones, tablets, and multifunctional devices, which have been instrumental in increasing access to healthcare.
- Providers are being challenged to explore new disease treatments and research findings in patients.
- In telemedicine, use of cardiac monitors in the ICU and telehealth skills in using monitoring devices in home health care are examples of other areas that are growing rapidly in high-tech healthcare.

Some of the pending technologies that will impact patients, clinical nurses, INs, and healthcare consumers include:

- New methods of medication administration
- New monitoring devices and miniaturization of devices in the home that can collect data such as measuring devices in the bathroom
- Wearable computing devices such as sensors embedded in clothing to track activities of an Alzheimer's patient.
- Sensors embedded throughout an apartment to monitor those in senior living apartments called smart apartments.

These are just a few examples of research and development occurring today. All of the examples discussed here require the knowledge and skills of an NI or someone with extensive knowledge and experience in informatics to explain and facilitate utilization and functionality to both information technologists (IT) and clinical nurses in practice (Box 2.1).

BOX 2.1

ROLES OF THE INFORMATICS NURSE: SELECTED ESSENTIALS

With EHR implementations	• Conduct workflow/gap analyses. • Prioritize data-collection activities in order to analyze data for reports; use analytical models, algorithms, and other tools for assessment and evaluation. • Demonstrate and be able to differentiate among and apply tools to collect outcomes information. • Participate in planning and contribute to teams during the design, implementation, and evaluation of information systems.
Roles in clinical practice	• Use of smartphones, tablets, and multifunctional devices • Telemedicine—cardiac monitors in ICU • Telehealth monitoring devices in home health

QSEN SCENARIO

You are a member of a medical–surgical team that is about to be included in the selection of the new EHR system that will be implemented at your organization over the next six months.

Which of the roles would you assume as an informatics nurse, as a team member, or as the clinical nurse?

▧ Questions to Consider Before Reading On

1. *List three NI organizations. Can any nurse join these organizations?*
2. *Discuss the purpose of the organizations in supporting NI members and all nurses. What are some of the benefits of the organizations?*

▧ Professional Informatics Organizations for Role Support and Career Development

There are many multidisciplinary and NI specialty groups whose key focus is using informatics to support and improve healthcare through the application of information and technology to practice. A partial list of these professional organizations includes the American Nursing Informatics Association (ANIA), International Medical Informatics Association (IMIA), Healthcare Information and Management Systems Society (HIMSS), American Health Information Management Association (AHIMA), and the Alliance for Nursing Informatics (ANI). This list is not inclusive but contains the most frequently referenced groups noted as supporting the competency development and education of informatics nurses as well as providing basic education opportunities for all practicing nurses through the presentation of webinars and other continuing-education-unit (CEU) opportunities (Box 2.2). An additional important organization to mention is Sigma Theta Tau International (STTI); it offers information and support for NI.

The ANIA provides many opportunities for members to obtain CEUs on a monthly basis as well as to present at annual conferences. It also provides NI certification courses for members who wish to become certified—these courses are held throughout the year and at national conferences. CEUs can be applied to maintain continuing education for licenses. Members also receive the *Computer, Informatics Nursing (CIN)* journal.

The AHIMA was formed by the American College of Surgeons to improve clinical records. Today, clinical and hospital data have expanded well beyond use by a single hospital to many within an enterprise. AHIMA offers credentialing programs in health information management, coding, and healthcare privacy and security programs.

The Alliance of Nursing Informatics (ANI) untied many of the local smaller nursing informatics groups and is sponsored by the American Medical Informatics Association (AMIA) and the HIMSS (Alliance for Nursing Informatics, 2014; Healthcare Information and Management Systems Society, 2014), which included AMIA when it first started. Today, membership is offered through the main group and dues are collected so the organization can provide education and role-competency development programs and support all NI initiatives. ANI membership includes membership in the working groups: ANIA, AMIA, and HIMSS. There are also a number of international informatics organizations that are not listed here. Overall, most NI-related organizations have nursing working groups within a multidisciplinary membership, as well as a specific focus on NI, such as AMIA.

The STTI supports all nurses in education, knowledge, and professional development to make a difference in health worldwide. It also offers a special leadership award given to an informatics expert whose contributions improve quality, safety, outcomes, and decision-making in health and nursing, nationally and internationally.

BOX 2.2

PROFESSIONAL INFORMATICS ORGANIZATIONS

Alliance for Nursing Informatics (ANI)	Sponsored by AMIA and HIMSS; provides a unified voice for nursing informatics
American Health Information Management Association (AHIMA)	Offers credentialing programs in health information management, coding, and healthcare privacy and security

(continued)

BOX 2.2 (*continued*)

American Nursing Informatics Association (ANIA)	Provides educational and CEU opportunities and nursing informatics certification preparation seminars
Healthcare Information and Management Systems Society (HIMSS)	An international organization that promotes a better understanding of healthcare information and management systems, as the acronym indicates
International Medical Informatics Association (IMIA)	A scientific organization that promotes informatics in healthcare and biomedical and informatics research and education

CEU, continuing-education units.

CASE SCENARIO

Tanya has been a nurse for 10 years in neurology critical care and is hearing more and more about the new discipline of NI. She is beginning to explore the discipline to determine exactly what it is and is asking questions of her managers and coworkers. She hears back from some coworkers who state, "it is just a type of data collection" and they tell Tanya that she would not enjoy it because it will "take her away from the nursing she loves."

Her manager refers her to the new IN just hired by the hospital to help with the implementation of a new EHR system that will be implemented soon.

Tanya agrees to start exploring the NI discipline with the new IN to find out exactly what the IN does.

Two of the first questions Tanya asks are:

1. How is NI different from what I currently do as a bedside nurse taking care of patients in the neurology ICU?

2. What kind and what type of skills are needed in NI? I am not excited about just collecting and analyzing data.

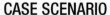 Questions to Consider Before Reading On

1. *What do you currently understand about the nursing theories that support NI? Are any of the same theories also applicable to other types of nurses? If so, name three that apply to all nurses.*

2. *What are the components of DIKW?*

3. *Discuss the differences among Benner's levels of proficiency: novice, advanced beginner, and competent.*

■ Theories That Contribute to Nursing Informatics' Competency, Skills, and Practice

Nursing theory facilitates the development of nursing knowledge and provides principles to support all nursing practice. Theory shapes practice and provides a method for expressing key ideas regarding the principles of nursing practice (Walker & Avant, 2011). Nursing theory is developed from groups of concepts and describes their interrelationships, thus presenting a systematic view of nursing-related events. The purpose of theory is to describe, explain, predict, and/or prescribe (Chinn & Kramer, 2011; Reed & Shearer, 2007; Risjord, 2009; Walker & Avant, 2011). The theories that contribute to nursing informatics competencies, skills, and practice are summarized in Box 2.4.

Different levels of nursing theory exist; these levels include metatheory, grand theory, and mid-range theories. Metatheories focus on theory about theory. These theories develop through asking philosophical and methodological questions to form a nursing foundation. Grand theories give a broad perspective for the purpose and structure of nursing practice (Peterson & Bredow, 2008; Walker & Avant, 2011). One of the greatest contributions are grand theories, largely developed between 1960 and the 1980s, provides for nursing through the differentiation between nursing and medical practice. In contrast, mid-range nursing theories contain a related set of ideas and variables, are narrower in scope, and are testable (Smith & Liehr, 2008; Walker & Avant, 2011). Regardless of the theory level, it is important for all nurses to understand nursing theories as they provide the foundation for practice.

The Data–Information–Knowledge–Wisdom (DIKW) Framework

The initial model evaluated for use in NI was the DIKW framework, which originated from the computer informatics and information sciences, particularly knowledge management (Blum, 1986). The data–information–knowledge portion of the framework was first discussed in nursing in Graves and Corcoran's (1989) work; the DIKW framework—*wisdom* was added—was first described for use in NI by Nelson (2002) and adopted by the ANA in 2008 (ANA, 2008; Schleyer & Beaudry, 2009; Thompson & Warren, 2009).

The DIKW components consist of four overlapping concepts—data, information, knowledge, and wisdom—listed with examples of how they might apply to NI.

- Data are symbols that represent objects, events, and their environments, which alone have little meaning. Examples are numbers, raw data such as 1, 2, 3, 4, 5.

- Information is data that has been given structure. Example: Data (numbers) defined as a blood pressure (BP) reading have meaning—120/80 mmHg.

- Knowledge is derived by discovering patterns and relationships between types of information (Nelson, 2002). What does 120/80 mmHg mean in the context of BP—is it too high, low, or normal?

- Wisdom is using knowledge correctly to handle or explain human problems. The ANA describes *wisdom* as the ability to evaluate the information and knowledge within the context of caring and use judgment to make care decisions (ANA, 2008; Matney, Brewster, Sward, Cloyes, & Staggers, 2011). For example, what do you do with a BP of 120/80 mmHg?

The DIKW model has been widely adopted in NI. Two key questions should be considered: (1) Does DIKW serve clinical information systems, nurses, and NIs or all three? and (2) what level of theory does DIKW occupy? The DIKW model has been valuable in advancing the independent field of NI by providing a framework for what data are and how data are applied (Matney, Avant, & Staggers, 2015; Ronquillo, Currie, & Rodney, 2016).

The response to question #1 is that DIKW serves all three because nurses and NIs are the users of the clinical information systems that retrieve and input data and patient information. The answer to the second question is less clear.

Benner: Novice-to-Expert Model

One of the best known nursing practice models is Benner's model: From Novice to Expert. In 1989, Dreyfus and Dreyfus (1980) created the Dreyfus model, which suggests that in the acquisition and development of a skill, one passes through five levels of proficiency: novice, advanced beginner, competent, proficient, to become an expert. Benner (1982, 2004) adapted the model to explain how nursing students and professional nurses acquire nursing skills, including NI. For example, a novice follows rules provided for each situation and is not flexible; at the competent stage, there he or she can better differentiate between what is and what is not important while applying perspectives; with proficiency, decision are made using intuition based on past experiences; and finally, the expert intuitively understands a situation and immediately connects an action to this understanding (Ajay, 2003). The five stages as defined by Benner are presented here.

- *Novice*: Level I. Novice beginners have no experience with the circumstances in which they are expected to perform tasks. In order to give novice beginners access to experience with patients, they are taught in terms of goals and objectives. These goals are features of the task that can be recognized without situational experience. Common attributes accessible to the novice include taking weights, measuring intake and output, and recording temperature, BP, pulse, and other such measurable parameters.

- *Advanced Beginner*: Level II. The advanced beginner can demonstrate marginally acceptable performance. This person has coped with enough real situations to note (or to have them pointed out by a mentor) the recurrent meaningful situational components, called *aspects*, such as assessing patient/learner readiness.

- *Competent*: Level III. Is typified by the nurse who has been on the job two to three years, develops when the nurse begins to see their actions in terms of long-range goals. Competence is evidenced by the fact that the nurse begins to see their actions in terms of long-range goals or plans.

- *Proficient*: Level IV. With continued practice, the nurse moves to the proficient stage. Characteristically, the proficient performer perceives situations as wholes, rather than in terms of one view, and performance is guided by principles. Experience teaches the proficient nurse typical events to expect in a given situation and how to modify plans in response to these.

- *Expert:* Level V. At the expert level, the nurse no longer relies on an analytical principle (rule, guideline) to connect their understanding of the situation to an appropriate action. The expert nurse, with enormous background of experience, has an intuitive grasp of the situation and zeros in on the accurate region of the problem (Benner, 2004). An example of what this process might look like is shown in Figure 2.1.

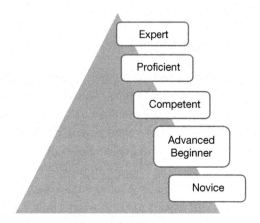

FIGURE 2.1 Adaptation of Benner's model: Novice to Expert.

SOURCE: Sipes (2018).

Questions to Consider Before Reading On

1. *Which of the theories or models described here are you most familiar with?*

2. *As you review the theories described in the next section, consider how you would apply a specific model or theory to your current practice.*

3. *Why is it important to understand theories? How do they support your clinical practice?*

Chaos Theory

Chaos theory was first discussed in 1963 by meteorologist Edward Lorenz, who attemped to predict weather using established equations. Chaos theory is associated with the butterfly effect, a theory that states that a small change can result in a significant effect later. The butterfly effect was initially used with weather prediction and states that when a butterfly moves its wings, this movement can cause a tornado in another part of the world. The flapping of the butterfly's wings have the capacity to create tiny changes in the atmosphere that lead to violent weather conditions elsewhere on the planet. The butterfly effect deals with things that are effectively impossible to predict or control, such as the rapid growth of technology, the NI specialty, weather, the stock market, to name a few. In plain language, the butterfly effect says that tiny changes within a complex system, such as an information system, can lead to results that are impossible to predict.

Chaos theory deals with differences in outcomes that depend on the conditions present at the starting point. Chaos theory, similar to general systems theory, addresses a structure without reducing it to its basic parts. This makes it useful with information systems, which are very complex. In summary, chaos theory says that what appears to be chaotic really has an underlying order in which initial conditions influence experiences and events. Understanding that one process does not always follow another in a stepwise progression will stimulate new thinking.

If you have been involved in the implementation of a new EHR at a healthcare facility, you might have seen how the plan in place at the beginning of the process changed and did not result in the original planned outcome in the end—the plan changed over time as more information about the system and analysis of nursing workflows became available.

General Systems Theory

General systems theory is important to understand as it provides the foundation for how computer and other systems work, presented in Chapters 3 and 4: Hardware and Software. Von Bertalanffy (1973), a biologist, introduced the original theory, developed as a reaction against reducing events and experiences into smaller parts. In systems theory the focus is on the interaction among the various parts of the system instead of recognizing each individual part, considering the whole greater than the sum of its parts.

For example, when you use a computer to document/input patient information, what if that information just stayed there and did not go anywhere for other providers to access? What if you only completed a patient assessment and took if no further, meaning you offered no diagnosis, did not anticipate outcomes, or plan further—you only focused on the "smaller parts" and not the whole?

As you will learn in Chapter 4: Hardware, systems are either a closed or open and maintained by a feedback loop. A closed system might be the circulatory system. An open system interacts with other components as shown in the example that follows. Every living organism is essentially an open system. Negative feedback results when there is a lack of something—positive feedback occurs when there is too much of something. There is a feedback loop that functions on input, throughput, and output. Input involves adding information to the system, process (throughput) where the system preforms using the input and passes through, output is the results of the process. Consider the steps in this process as you might when "inputting" a medication order (Figure 2.2).

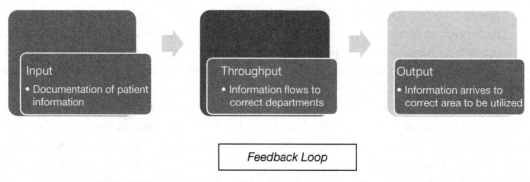

FIGURE 2.2 Adaptations of the General Systems Theory model.

SOURCE: Sipes (2018).

Other nursing theories based on Von Bertalanffy's General Systems theory include:

- Neuman's Systems Theory, Rogers's Theory of Unitary Human Beings
- Roy's Adaptation Model
- Imogene King's Theory of Goal Attainment
- Orem's Self-Care Deficit Theory
- Johnson's Behavior Systems Model

■ Questions to Consider Before Reading On

1. *Are any of the theorists and theories described familiar to you?*
2. *Have you reviewed and applied any of these to your current practice, for example, the change theory?*

Cognitive Science

Cognitive science is the study of the mind, intelligence, and how we think (Thagard, 2010) and looks at processes and mental activities. Cognitive technologies include computers, smartphones, web browsers and media that we use to help learning and memory and problem solving in today's high-tech world—both at work and in daily life. Cognitive science provides the framework for designing tools to support computer and screen development, for example; understanding the steps for constructive use of information and information processing to gain knowledge (Staggers & Thompson, 2002). This is a basic description of cognitive science. How do you think understanding this can influence your practice?

Computer Science

Computer science is the study of algorithms used to solve computation problems by using the computer as the tool that defines and connects the steps. If it is determined that a problem can be solved by developing and using an algorithm, then an automated solution to the problem can be built by an analyst. Once this is determined, a machine/computer program can be built to generate the solution. Why do you think it is important to know some of the basics of this theory?

Change Theory

Lewin's change theory provides a framework for managing change, most frequently seen with changes that come with the implementation of an EHR. It has three stages—unfreezing, change, refreezing, as well as three major concepts: driving forces, restraining forces, and equilibrium. Driving forces are those that push in a direction that causes change to occur such as in healthcare leadership. They facilitate change because they push the organization in a desired direction. They cause a shift in the equilibrium toward change.

Restraining forces are those forces that counter the driving forces. They hinder change because they push the organization in the opposite direction. They cause a shift in the equilibrium that opposes change. Equilibrium is a state of being in which driving forces equal restraining forces, and no change occurs. It can be raised or lowered by changes that occur between the driving and restraining forces (Barrow & Toney-Butler, 2018).

Lewin's stages of change include (1) identifying a need to change (unfreezing), (2) implementing change (moving), and (3) achieving a state of balance (refreezing), which applies to implementing the final project (Mitchell, 2018).

- Unfreezing is a process that involves finding a method of making it possible for people to let go of an old pattern that was somehow counterproductive. It is necessary to overcome the strains of individual resistance and group conformity.

- There are three methods that can lead to the achievement of unfreezing. The first is to increase the driving forces that direct behavior away from the existing situation or status quo. Second, decrease the restraining forces that negatively affect the movement from the existing equilibrium. Third, find a combination of the first two methods.

- The change stage, which is also called *moving to a new level* or *movement*, involves a process of change in thoughts, feeling, behaviors, or all three that is in some way liberating or more productive than what came before.

- The refreezing stage is establishing the change as the new habit, so that it now becomes the "standard operating procedure." Without this final stage, it can be easy to go back to old habits (Figure 2.3).

Lewin's Three-Stage Change Process — Practical
Steps

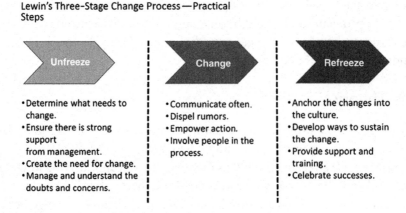

FIGURE 2.3 Lewin's Change Model.

SOURCE: Mulholland, B. (2017). 8 critical change management models to evolve and survive. Retrieved from https://www.process.st/change-management-models.

Diffusion of Innovation Theory

Another important theory is Roger's diffusion of innovation theory, which explores leaders, followers, and how the media can influence opinion leaders and followers. According to Rogers (2010), personal characteristics influence whether people adopt an innovation rapidly. Based on the adopters' characteristics, adopters can be divided into five categories that follow a bell-shaped curve.

- The first 2.5% of individuals in a system who adopt an innovation are called *innovators*; they are the pioneers with the most courage to accept the innovation.

- The next 13.5%, called *early adopters*, are the stakeholders in a social system and usually lead people to change. They seek information and advice from the pioneers, and their acceptance behavior is the most appropriate endorsement of the innovations.

- The third group, named the *early majority*, occupies the area between 1 standard deviation and the median under the curve; people in this group are on higher alert and have interest in new ideas, but adopt these ideas after others' successful experiences. They mainly learn from their close associates and rely on personal communication channels to diffuse the innovation. They are more risk averse than early adopters, and they will take a longer time to evaluate all possibilities before accepting the innovation.

- The fourth group, named the *late majority*, adopts the innovation after the left half of the population under the curve does. They are usually more conservative, cautious, and suspicious, even though the innovation has been safely tried by most of the early majority and early adopters. The main reasons for the delay in adoption are the uncertainties and caution caused by limited resources or inadequate information.

■ The last group is named *laggards*. They are conservatives or vulnerable groups with the fewest resources, limited information and unstable incomes, or are isolated from the social support system. They fall behind due to the neglect of social system (Rogers, 2010).

BOX 2.3

REFLECTION—DIFFUSION OF INNOVATIONS AND CHANGE THEORY

When you read the diffusion of innovation information on change, reflect on a change that you experienced at some point in your career or college program. As you learned new ideas, consider:

1. How did that occur?
2. Can you relate the changes you experienced to this theory—the diffusion of innovations?
3. Which group were you in?

Change theory is another important theory proposed by Lewin as discussed earlier. Change theory describes a three-phase process in which we open our minds, deal with the change, and adapt to the change. It is important to understand the dynamics at work when dealing with change and expecting others to deal with change also.

Think about different reactions to the change:

1. Can you trace the phases described by Lewin?
2. How have you dealt with change?

CASE SCENARIO

Brian is on a team that has just been told today that they will be implementing a new EHR system over the next 6 months. His role as a nursing informaticist is to first support and define the workflows for all of the nursing staff, then identify the gaps that the new system will address.

Some of his coworkers in the meeting express negative comments regarding what they have heard about how these systems do not work and said they are not in favor of these changes.

Brian is considering how to present the benefits in a positive way to the team so team members will better accept the upcoming changes:

1. What other barriers should Brian anticipate?
2. What suggestions should he apply from both change theory and Roger's diffusion theory to help address the barriers he will experience?
3. What stages of change are his coworkers in now?

BOX 2.4

THEORIES THAT CONTRIBUTE TO NURSING INFORMATICS

THEORY/MODEL	CONTRIBUTION
Benner: Novice to Expert	A five-stage model indicating how people advance from novice to expert with education and experience. For NI, the advancement moves from basic to advanced computer skills and experienced to developed expertise.
Change	When applied to a situation, change theory improves one's chances of success with an EHR implementation when expectations are shared by all.
Chaos	Consideration of small changes that occur at the starting point of an event can lead to differences in outcomes, such as how medications might be documented in the new EHR.
Cognitive science	Understanding the mind improves memory and the ability to gain knowledge from an information system such as a smartphone; cognitive science is part of the field of social informatics.
Computer science	The IN will use technology and informatics to apply algorithms so as to analyze the steps in a problem, thereby gaining knowledge, after which automation is used to solve problems.
Diffusion of innovation (Rogers)	People go through stages when deciding to adopt an innovation such as an EHR; the stages are innovators, early adopters, early majority, late majority, and laggards.
Data–information knowledge–wisdom (DIKW)—a NI theory	DIKW provides a perspective on nursing data, information, and knowledge—key components of NI—used to manage and communicate nursing information in healthcare. Wisdom is the highest level of application of knowledge.
General systems	This theory provides insight into the complexity of an information system by breaking things down into smaller parts in order to better understand a process to see how one might affect the other. For NI, if documenting a patient care note, understanding where the note goes so everyone can see it is important. Or if a medication were given, then documented, but did not show up in the right area, it would be important to know why and where the process was "broken."

EHR, electronic health record; IN, informatics nurse; NI, nurse informatics.

Critical Thinking Questions and Activities

- *As you review the informatics roles listed previously, how do these apply to what you currently know and practice?*

- *Conducting an Internet search on NI, what are some of the other roles you might be interested in? What are some examples in your organization?*

- *As you review the benefits of the different informatics organizations, which one would you join? Why?*

- *Which stage of Benner's model are you currently in? What are your future plans with regard to advancing stages?*

SUMMARY

This chapter continued to provide key components that comprise the foundations of NI. Readers were introduced to organizations that provide support and education about what NI is and offered skills to use to develop the IN role if that is the career path chosen. Discussion, definitions, and the differences between a skill and competency were provided as were reasons why it is important to develop these in your practice. Selected roles were identified and explained with examples based on the AACN Essentials defined in Chapter 1. Models and theories with examples and diagrams that apply to all nursing practice and to NI specifically, were provided.

The ANA (2015b) *Nursing Informatics: Scope and Standards of Practice*—standards 8 and 9—were addressed using this content.

- Standard 8: The NI addresses the need for education, attaining knowledge and competence reflecting current nursing practice. Competency example: Demonstrates commitment to lifelong learning.

- Standard 9: The NI integrates evidence and research into practice. Competency example: Demonstrates application of and integration of evidence and research into practice.

Although these standards list specific information related to NI, they are relevant to all practicing nurses.

References

Ajay, B. (2003). Student profiling: The Dreyfus model revisited. *Education for Primary Care, 14*(3), 360.

Alliance for Nursing Informatics. (2014). Homepage. Retrieved from http://www.allianceni .org

American Nurses Association. (2008). *Nursing informatics: Scope and standards of practice.* Silver Spring, MD: Author.

American Nurses Association. (2015a). Health IT initiatives (pp. 1–2, 190). Retrieved from http:// nursingworld.org/MainMenuCaterfories/ThePracticeofProfessional Nursing/Health-IT.org

American Nurses Association. (2015b). *Nursing informatics: Scope and standards of practice.* (2nd ed.). Silver Spring, MD: Author.

Barrow, J. M., & Toney-Butler, T. J. (2018). *Change, management.* Treasure Island, FL: StatPearls Publishing. Retrieved from https://www.ncbi.nlm.nih.gov/books/NBK459380

Benner, P. (1982). From novice to expert. *American Journal of Nursing, 82*(3), 402–407.

Benner, P. (2004). Using the Dreyfus model of skill acquisition to describe and interpret skill acquisition and clinical judgment in nursing practice and education. *Bulletin of Science, Technology and Society, 24*(3), 188–199. doi:10.1177/0270467

Blum, B. L. (Ed.). (1986). *Clinical information systems.* New York, NY: Springer Publishing.

Chinn, P. L., & Kramer, M. K. (2011). *Integrated theory and knowledge development in nursing* (8th ed.). St. Louis, MO: Elsevier Mosby.

Dreyfus, S., & Dreyfus, H. (1980). *A five stage model of the mental activities involved in directed skill acquisition.* Berkeley: California University Berkeley Operations Research Center.

Graves, J. R., & Corcoran, S. (1989). The study of nursing informatics. *Image, Journal of Nursing Scholarship, 21,* 227–231. doi:10.1111/j.1547-5069.1989.tb00148.x

Healthcare Information and Management Systems Society (HIMSS). (2014). Homepage. Retrieved from http://www/himss.org

Matney, S., Avant, K., & Staggers, N. (2015). Toward an understanding of wisdom in nursing. *OJIN: The Online Journal of Issues in Nursing, 21*(1), 7. doi:10.3912/OJIN.Vol21No01PPT02

Matney, S., Brewster, P., Sward, K., Cloyes, K., & Staggers, N. (2011). Philosophical approaches to the nursing informatics data–information–knowledge–wisdom framework. *ANS. Advances in Nursing Science, 34*(1), 6–18. doi:10.1097/ANS.0b013e3182071813

Mitchell, G. (2018). Selecting the best theory to implement planned change. *Nursing Management, 20,* 32–37. doi:10.7748/nm2013.04.20.1.32.e1013

Mulholland, B. (2017). Eight critical change management models to evolve and survive. Retrieved from https://www.process.st/change-management-models

Nelson, R. (2002). Major theories supporting health care informatics. In S. Englebardt & R. Nelson (Eds.), *Health care informatics: An interdisciplinary approach* (pp. 3–27). St. Louis, MO: Mosby.

Peterson, S. J., & Bredow, T. S. (2008). *Middle range theories: Application to nursing research.* Philadelphia, PA: Lippincott Williams & Wilkins.

Pillar, B., & Golumbic, N. (Eds.). (1993). Acquiring and delivering knowledge from and for patient care. In B. Pillar & N. Golumbic (Eds.) *Nursing informatics: Enhancing patient care* (p. 12). Bethesda, MD: National Center for Nursing Research, U.S. Department of Health and Human Services.

Reed, P. G., & Shearer, N. C. (2007). *Perspectives on nursing theory* (5th ed.). Philadelphia, PA: Lippincott Williams & Wilkins.

Risjord, M. W. (2009). *Nursing knowledge: Science, practice, and philosophy.* West Sussex, UK: Wiley-Blackwell.

Rogers, E. M. (2010). *Diffusion of innovations* (4th ed.). New York, NY: Simon and Schuster.

Ronquillo, C., Currie, L., & Rodney, P. (2016). The evolution of data-information-knowledge -wisdom in nursing informatics. *Advances in Nursing Science, 39*(1), E1–E18. doi:10.1097/ANS.0000000000000107

Schleyer, R., & Beaudry, S. (2009). Data to wisdom: Informatics in telephone triage nursing practice. *AAACN Viewpoint, 31*(5), 1, 10–13.

Smith, M. J., & Liehr, P. R. (2008). *Middle range theory for nursing.* New York, NY: Springer Publishing.

Staggers, N., & Thompson, C. B. (2002). The evolution of definitions for nursing informatics: A critical analysis and revised definition. *Journal of the American Medical Informatics Association: JAMIA, 9(3), 255–261.* http://doi.org/10.1197/jamia.M0946

Systems Theory in Nursing; Current Nursing. (2012). Systems Theory in Nursing. Retrieved from http://currentnursing.com/nursing_theory/systems_theory_in_nursing.html

Thagard, P. (2010). *The brain and the meaning of life*. Princeton, NJ: Princeton University Press.

Thompson, T. L., & Warren, J. J. (2009). Are they all data? Understanding the work of organizational knowledge. *Clinical Nurse Specialist, 23*(4), 185–186. doi:10.1097/NUR.0b0 13e3181aae374

von Bertalanffy, L. (1968). *General system theory: Foundations, development, applications*. New York, NY: George Braziller.

von Bertalanffy, L. (1973). *Perspectives on general system theory*. E. Taschdjian (Ed.). New York, NY: George Braziller.

Walker, L. O., & Avant, K. C. (2011). *Strategies for theory construction in nursing* (5th ed.). Upper Saddle River, NJ: Pearson. Retrieved from https://monoskop.org/images/7/77/Von _Bertalanffy_Ludwig_General_System_Theory_1968.pdf

PART II

NURSING INFORMATICS: ESSENTIAL COMPUTER CONCEPTS

CHAPTER 3

NURSING INFORMATICS: FIRST THINGS FIRST—HARDWARE

CAROLYN SIPES

LEARNING OBJECTIVES AND OUTCOMES

Upon completion of this chapter, the reader will be able to:

- Discuss essential hardware components of a computer.
- Describe basic operations of the central processing unit (CPU).
- Describe what common computer input, output, and storage devices are and how they apply to your practice.
- Describe computer network hardware devices and their functions.
- Discuss why it is important to understand the basics of computer hardware and its functionality. Describe how it impacts your daily practice.
- Discuss other ways you use a computer.

⊙ KEY NURSING INFORMATICS TERMS

Some of the key concepts and terms you will hear in the discipline of nursing informatics are:

Arithmetic logic unit (ALU)	"Gooey" (GUI)
Cache	Hardware
Central processing unit (CPU)	Input
Flash drive (thumb drive)	Kilobyte (KB)
Gigabyte (GB)	Megabyte (MB)

⊙ KEY NURSING INFORMATICS TERMS (*continued*)

Motherboard	Software
Operating system (OS)	Storage devices
Output	Terabyte (TB)
Peripherals	Throughput
Random access memory (RAM)	Universal Serial Bus (USB)
Read-only memory (ROM)	Workstations on wheels (WOWs)

INTRODUCTION: COMPUTER COMPONENTS—HARDWARE

You may already understand some basics of an information system including "computer hardware," which means all of the physical components of a computer. As most people have a computer, you may not even know someone who has neither a computer nor any other technical device. Your role as a nurse has probably become much more complex as newer technology and devices are introduced to your everyday practice. This may include new infusion pumps, ICU equipment such as cardiac and other monitors, and especially computers everywhere. You may ask: What else do I need to know about a computer, its parts, and how it functions?

The concept of computer science, one of the building blocks of nursing informatics (NI), was introduced in Chapter 2. This chapter will provide an overview of the main hardware components of a computer such as operations of the central processing unit (CPU), as well as input, output, and storage devices, to name a few. With today's advancing and more complex technology, it is important to have a basic understanding of the tools and technology you use to provide high-quality and safer patient care. The basic skills needed to become proficient in using technology are known as the "NI skills, competencies, and knowledge." Using NI skills coupled with advanced technology will help you become a better nurse. Understanding some basics of computer hardware not only impacts your current practice but will also influence other uses and understanding such as gaming.

▓ Questions to Consider Before Reading On

1. *What is computer hardware?*
2. *What is RAM?*
3. *What is ROM?*
4. *What is the main purpose of the motherboard?*
5. *List three computer devices.*

Essential Computer Hardware Basics

In Chapter 1 of this text you have already learned what NI is, how the TIGER initiative and the IOM report influenced and pushed the critical need for and advancement of learning computer skills and competencies in order to practice in today's high-technology-driven healthcare environments. History and evolution of NI was presented as well as expectations of why you need to develop competencies in order to practice in today's high-tech healthcare environment in order to improve patient care.

All computers require what is known as the "operating system" (OS) in order to work. The computer is a tool with the main purpose of processing data and information (input), storing and retrieving data (throughput), and providing (output) the data to the end-user.

The total type of processing depends on the programs or applications (apps) loaded on the computer that direct the functions. The concepts of input, throughput, and output were introduced in Chapter 2 in General Systems Theory with an example of what the process flow is (see Chapter 2).

This is an important concept to understand as this is how you access your email. The apps work with a specific OS but only certain applications will work on a specific OS. For example, there are apps that will work on Microsoft Windows—the most common OS—and not on a Mac OSX, Linux, or Google Chrome OS.

Previously, computers used a disk OS (DOS) where the screens were black with white text—not very user-friendly and difficult to read. Today computers have come a long way—today, the point-and-click system is known as a "graphical user interface" or GUI (pronounced "gooey").

Questions to Consider Before Reading On

1. *Discuss the process flow of information and data into and out of the computer.*
2. *What is the main purpose of the CPU?*
3. *What is the main component of a computer?*
4. *What are the four main processes of information flow in a computer?*

Basic Computer Hardware

The part of the main architecture of a computer includes the internal components such as the electronic circuits, microchips and processors, CPU, motherboard, random access memory (RAM), read-only memory (ROM), and graphic and sound cards. These are attached to an internal component called a "motherboard."

The main component of the computer is the motherboard where the electric lines are soldered and desgined in such a way that data can flow across. As noted in Box 3.1, the motherboard contains the microchips including the CPU and other wiring. The motherboard also is the place for memory storage and retreival. The ROM stores permanent information that allows the computer to start or "boot up." ROM is where programs are stored that control the CPU, which provides ovesight for computer functions.

BOX 3.1

PROCESS FLOW OF INFORMATION—INPUT AND OUTPUT TO DEVICES

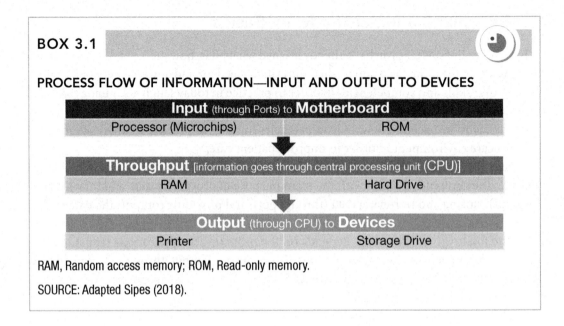

RAM, Random access memory; ROM, Read-only memory.

SOURCE: Adapted Sipes (2018).

Figure 3.1 gives an example of a motherboard and its components. The CPU is sometimes known as the "brain," "processor," or "microprocessor" of the computer; it controls the operation of all parts of the computer; it is a small square with short pins as connectors on the underside attached to the motherboard. It is responsible for executing a sequence of stored instructions, or programs, and is responsible for interpreting and performing all types of data- processing operations. It stores data, transitional results, and instructions (program). It performs most of the commands from the computer's other hardware and software. Many devices use a CPU, including desktop, laptop, tablet computers, and smartphones, as well as a flat-screen television set.

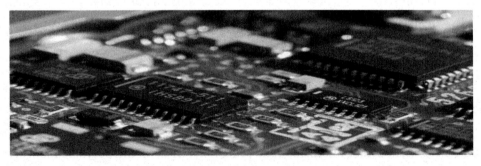

FIGURE 3.1 Motherboard of computer—contains circuits where main electronics of computer are plugged in.

A CPU with which you might be most familiar is Intel—a sticker on your laptop. For example, it might list it as Intel inside, CORE 17 vPro, which tells the version of the CPU in your computer.

The very simple explanation for the process of data and information flow in the computer is that information flows in though ports to the motherboard where the processor or microchips and ROM are attached containing the circuits where the main electronics of the computer can be found.

There are also two sections known as an "arithmetic and logic unit" (ALU), which is a complex digital circuit. You need this to be able to perform arithmetical and logical operations. Arithmetical sections perform arithmetical operations such as addition, subtraction, multiplication, and division. You may have noticed you have a calculator listed under the applications on your computer. The logic unit is responsible for performing logical operations such as comparing, selecting, matching, and merging of different data or information. The ALU is the major part of the computer system that handles different calculations. Depending on the design of the ALU, it makes the CPU more powerful and efficient.

There are other devices in the computer case that are not part of the main architecture of the systems discussed earlier, such as the cooling system, universal serial bus (usb) connectors, and other tools. the computer is a tool with the main purpose of processing data and information (input), storing and retrieving data (throughput), and providing (output) the data to the end-user. the total type of processing depends on the programs loaded on the computer that direct the function.

▧ Questions to Consider Before Reading On

1. *What is the purpose of RAM? How would you use it? What can happen to data if you try to store it here?*
2. *What is the purpose of ROM?*
3. *What is the function of Cache?*
4. *What are the three main types of computer memory?*

Main Memory

What is memory? The size of memory is very important to understand as it determines how much work your computer can control. Main memory or RAM is the internal memory of the CPU for storing data, programs, and program results. It is a read/write memory which stores access time in RAM and is independent of the address, that is, each storage location inside the memory is as easy to reach as other locations and takes the same amount of time. Data in the RAM can be accessed randomly. RAM is volatile, that is, data stored in it are lost when we switch off the computer or if there is a power failure.

A smaller form of RAM is Cache, pronounced "cash," which speeds up processing by storing frequently used items in smaller units so that it can be accessed more quickly and reduce the amount of time it might take to search the larger RAM. By storing frequently used items/date/information in Cache it speeds up your access to information. If your computer is not "acting" correctly or too slowly—you will be asked by information technology (IT) or the Help Desk to clear your Cache.

Read-Only Memory

The memory from which we can only read but cannot write on it is called ROM. This type of memory is nonvolatile. The information is stored permanently in such memories during manufacture. ROM stores an instruction that is required to start a computer. Memory or storage can store instructions, data, and intermediate results. This unit supplies information to other units of the computer when needed. It is also known as "internal storage unit" or the "main memory" or the "primary storage" or "RAM." It stores the final results of processing before these results are released to an output device. All inputs and outputs are transmitted through the main memory. Its size affects speed, power, and capability. Primary memory and secondary memory are two types of memories in the computer.

Secondary Memory

This type of memory is also known as "external memory" or "nonvolatile memory." It is slower than the main memory and is used for storing data/information permanently. CPU directly does not access these memories; instead, they are accessed via input–output routines. The contents of secondary memories are first transferred to the main memory, and then the CPU can access it. For example, disk, CD-ROM, DVD, Flash or USB drives are removable and rewriteable devices and easily portable.

Now that you understand what memory is, a very important aspect of memory is the ability to store items such as pictures, which take up a lot of memory storage space. You may be asked to describe how large some of your text files or pictures might be if you are trying to email/send documents. You will need to describe those in "bytes." Some files may be too large to send depending on the receiver-end computer capabilities so you might have to divide the files into smaller bytes in order to send a file.

▨ Question to Consider Before Reading On

1. *What is the difference in the KB, MB, and TB?*

The following explains the main memory terms for storage units or the way information is stored (Box 3.2):

BOX 3.2

STORAGE UNITS AND DESCRIPTION TERMINOLOGY

Bit (Binary Digit): A binary digit is logical 0 and 1 representing a passive or an active state of a component in an electrical circuit.

Nibble: A group of 4 bits is called "nibble."

Byte: A group of 8 bits is called "byte." A byte is the smallest unit that can represent a data item or a character.

(continued)

BOX 3.2 (*continued*)

Word: A computer word, like a byte, is a group of fixed number of bits processed as a unit, which varies from computer to computer but is fixed for each computer.

The length of a computer word is called "word size" or "word length." It may be as small as 8 bits or as long as 96 bits. A computer stores the information in the form of computer words.

Box 3.3 lists terminology for larger storage units you may be familiar. These are the most common terms you may be familiar—this is only a partial listing as there are more. To see those you can explore the website www.lifewire.com.

BOX 3.3

STORAGE UNITS AND DESCRIPTION TERMINOLOGY

> Kilobyte (KB): 1 KB = 1,024 Bytes
> Megabyte (MB): 1 MB = 1,024 KB
> Gigabyte (GB): 1 GB = 1,024 MB
> Terabyte (TB): 1 TB = 1,024 GB
> Petabytes (PB): 1 PB = 1,024 TB

SOURCE: Fisher, T. (2018). Everything you need to know about computer hardware—Lifewire. https://www.lifewire.com.

CASE SCENARIO

Susan P. is a BSN student in her third year and has to purchase a new computer in order to effectively complete her studies since she has discovered her current computer is outdated and cannot be upgraded with newer, more efficient hardware. She also needs an upgraded, more powerful computer in order to work in a virtual learning environment (VLE) in order to complete some class assignments.

She is searching websites in order to gather more information regarding which personal computer (PC) will best suit her needs. She wants to understand more about how many bytes she will need for storage and RAM. Her friend, who also has a strong IT background, has suggested she review a number of websites that provide the recommendations for today's best resources.

(*continued*)

(continued)

> She starts to search the websites recommended but has a number of questions to answer first.
>
> 1. Will she be using it for gaming, which takes more power?
> 2. How many bytes will she need for storage?
> 3. How much bytes of RAM will she need?
> 4. How much will it cost since she is on a very limited budget?
> 5. How much battery life will be needed?

◾ Questions to Consider Before Reading On

1. *What components and peripherals should you have to enable you to work effectively in technology other than the basic computer components previously discussed? (See Figure 3.2).*
2. *Discuss what is involved in data processing.*
3. *What does output entail (See Box 3.4)?*

BOX 3.4

BASIC COMPUTER PROCESSES AND OPERATIONS

PROCESSES	EXPLANATION—WHAT OCCURS IN PROCESS
Input	Data entry and instructions for computer
Data storage	Saving and storing data to be utilized
Data processing	Performance of arithmetical and logical unit (ALU) operations on data—to convert to useful information
Output	The process of producing information or results, such as a printed report or visual display

---

CASE SCENARIO (CONTINUED)

Susan has decided on the computer that best meets her needs and now has questions about something described as "peripherals" she will need in order to complete any of her course assignments. As she begins to explore more about applications, she will need to understand more about the computer.

(continued)

(continued)

Questions she asks now include:

1. What is the definition of "peripheral"? Why do I need peripherals?

(She finds a diagram that will help explain what she needs to do now to set up her computer. She reviews the main *input peripherals* found in Figure 3.2.)

2. What other peripherals would I include in this list that I might use?

(She then reviews the main *output peripherals*.)

3. What other peripherals would I include in this list that I might use?

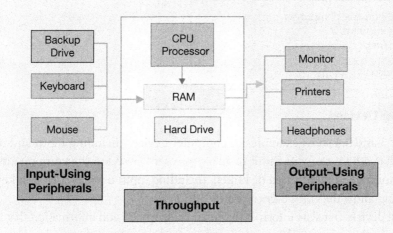

FIGURE 3.2 Basics of computer functionality diagram.

SOURCE: Sipes (2018).

▧ Questions to Consider Before Reading On

1. *What are three input devices you might use in your current practice?*
2. *What are three output devices you might use in your current practice?*
3. *Discuss the functionality of both input and output devices.*
4. *What are five main types of computers? Which would you use most frequently?*

Main Types of Computers

The computer is a tool with the main purpose of processing data and information (input), storing and retrieving data (throughput), and providing (output) the data to the end-user. The type of processing depends on the programs loaded on the computer that direct the function.

There are five basic types of computers. The general overview of the basic structures of a computer and their functionality and processes were discussed earlier. There is a category of special purpose computers that includes tablets, personal digital assistants (PDAs), and smartphones where utilization in healthcare facilities has exploded. In addition to the special purpose computers, there are four other basic types of computers: supercomputers with scientific applications that process huge amounts of information; mainframes that are fast, large, and process as well as store large amounts of information most frequently found in healthcare institutions; microcomputers (personal portable computers—PCs, notebooks, tablets) with which you are most familiar; and hand-held PCs/PDAs which have less functionality than the larger computers (Computer Hope, 2014; Domingo & Brant, 2017; Wagner & Bassett, 2017).

Summary: Five Main Types of Computers

- Special purpose computers
- Supercomputers
- Mainframes
- Microcomputers
- Hand-held PCs/PDAs

Computer Devices

Figures 3.3 and 3.4 show examples of computer devices including input and output devices. What others can you think of that you use? These are the components that can be seen, touched, and attached or linked, including input devices such as a keyboard or mouse, and allow the computer to receive input.

Output devices translate information into data, graphics, and information that is readable and usable by the end-user. These include a printer and monitor and secondary storage devices such as hard disks, CDs and DVDs, thumb drives (USB drives), earphones, microphones, and workstations on wheels (WOWs), sometimes referred to as "computers on wheels" (COWs), and the computer monitor. Can you think of other devices in your workplace that provide

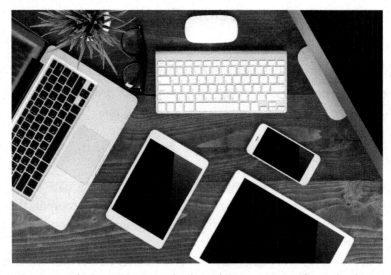

FIGURE 3.3 Computer devices: Computer keyboard, screen, smartphone, backup drive, tablet.

output of patient information such as IV pumps or ICU equipment/monitors?

Monitors, commonly called a "Visual Display Unit" (VDU), are the main output device of a computer. They form images from tiny dots, called "pixels," that are arranged in a rectangular form. The sharpness of the image depends upon the number of pixels. There are two kinds of viewing screen used for monitors (Fisher, 2018a, b). The most common monitor you will be familiar with is called a "flat-panel display monitor" that has reduced volume, weight, and power requirement in comparison to a much larger, older monitor you may also see in your workplace, called a "cathode ray tube" (CRT). You can hang them on walls or wear them on your wrists. Current uses of flat-panel displays include calculators, video games, monitors, laptop computers, and graphics displays. The example is what is most commonly seen now in the workplace (Fisher, 2018).

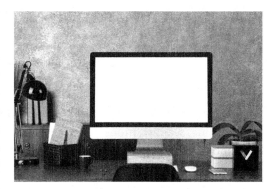

FIGURE 3.4 Computer monitor.

As you can see, there are many parts to an information system—the computer or "box" with all of the internal components and the external components such as the devices, also known as "peripherals."

In order to communicate effectively, including all documentation such as clinical charting, both hardware discussed here and software (discussed in Chapter 4) are needed to work together in order for the computer to work properly. The software will function only with the appropriate hardware and is the interface between the user and hardware.

QSEN SCENARIO

You want to download some information another nurse has shared with you as she hands you a thumb (flash) drive. What type of port would you use? Where would you find this on your computer?

Questions to Consider Before Reading On

1. *What are the two different types of ports?*
2. *For what is a port used?*

Connection Ports: A few words about ports. A port is a physical docking point where an external device can be connected to the computer, essentially a docking point through which information flows from a program to the computer or from the computer to a device such as a thumb drive. Ports are slots on the motherboard into which a cable of an external device or device such as a thumb drive is plugged. External devices discussed earlier can be connected to a computer using cables and ports, or simply just plugged in—examples might be the mouse, keyboard, and backup devices as well as other devices. There are two different types of ports:

- Serial Port: Used for external modems, and USB port
- Parallel Port: Used for scanners and printers

The USB port can connect all kinds of external USB devices such as an external hard disk, printer, scanner, mouse, and keyboard. Most computers provide two USB ports as a minimum. This is also where you would plug in a flash or thumb drive.

■ Critical Thinking Questions and Activities

When you review the Basic Information Process flow diagram in Box 3.4, list three of the input devices.

- *How are these attached to a computer? Where are these (ports) found on a computer?*

Using the same diagram in Box 3.4, list three output devices.

- *Where are these attached to a computer?*

You have learned about computers, how they work, and the peripherals needed in order to function as you need for school or home, whatever your need.

As you "build" your perfect computer now, what will you add as input devices and output devices? What OS will you be using?

After a review of functions needed on the new computer, such as storing large picture files, define how much memory you will need.

SUMMARY

You have reviewed the different types and parts of a computer and how the information flows into and out of a computer. Peripherals were defined as well as examples of what they are and their functions, which you may already know. This chapter provides an overview of large and small computers and devices. The concepts of data element size in terms of KB, MB, TB are explained including examples of why you need to understand this terminology and how it applies to your computer.

This chapter provided essential computer concepts and components including the hardware, which, in turn, provides the foundational understanding of computers and the relation to NI and information literacy and science. It provides examples of the main parts of a computer and how they function, integrating NI competencies and skills in order to link nurses to technology. With a better understanding of the computer basics, nurses can better grasp how to retrieve, organize, process, and manage data and information. The basics of computer software are provided in Chapter 4.

With this understating of computer basics with regard to hardware and functionality you are developing computer and information literacy and competencies with the application of the NI skills as well as developing informatics knowledge. The next chapter will tie in basics of software to hardware so you will understand how it all flows together.

References

Computer Hope. (2014). Computer Hope website. Retrieved from https://www.computerhope.com

Domingo, J., & Brant, T. (2017). The best desktop computers of 2018. *PC Magazine*. Retrieved from https://www.pcmag.com

Fisher, T. (2018a). Arithmetic Unit and Logic Unit (ALU). Retrieved from https://www.lifewire.com

Fisher, T. (2018b). Central Processing Unit (CPU). Retrieved from https://www.lifewire.com

Knapp, M. (2016). 9 key things to know before you buy a computer. Gear & Style Cheat Sheet. Retrieved from http://www.cheatsheet.com/technology/9-tips-for-picking-your-machine-computer-shopping-cheat-sheet.html

Knapp, M. (2017). 15 mistakes too many people make when buying a computer. Retrieved from https://www.cheatsheet.com/money-career/15-mistakes-too-many-people-make-when-buying-a-computer.html

Wagner, J., & Bassett, A. (2017). The best desktop computer you can buy: From hot rods to budget sleepers, our favorite desktops can handle anything. Retrieved from https://www.digitaltrends.com/computing/best-desktop-computers

CHAPTER 4

NURSING INFORMATICS: FIRST THINGS FIRST—SOFTWARE

JAMES SIPES | CAROLYN SIPES

LEARNING OBJECTIVES AND OUTCOMES

Upon completion of this chapter, the reader will be able to:

- Understand the differences between hardware and software.
- Discuss how software is applied in practice.
- List key software applications used in nursing clinical practice.
- Define differences between the Internet and World Wide Web.
- Discuss benefits of cloud computing and how they can be applied to clinical practice.
- Discuss steps to prevent malware attacks.
- Identify potential scenarios and examples of malware attacks and other security breaches.

⊙ KEY NURSING INFORMATICS TERMS

Some of the key concepts and terms you will hear in the discipline of nursing informatics are:

Application Software (apps)	Computer Literacy
Browsers	Computer Program
Cache	Computer Software
Cloud Computing and Services	Cookies

⊙ KEY NURSING INFORMATICS TERMS (*continued*)

Data Structures	Malware
Device Drivers	Operating System (OS)
Domains—Top Level	Routers
Internet	Utility Programs
Internet of Things (IoT)	Wide Area Network (WAN)
IP Address	Wi-Fi
Local Area Network (LAN)	World Wide Web (www)

INTRODUCTION: SOFTWARE

You may already know and understand the QSEN Knowledge, Skills, and Attitudes (KSAs) from Chapter 1 and have been applying them to your practice—but you may not understand how they fit into informatics. According to Cronenwett, Sherwood, Pohl, et al. (2009), the skills listed here are already practiced by most RN-to-BSN students. You have the skills to:

- Navigate the electronic health record (EHR)
- Document and plan patient care in an EHR
- Use communication technologies to coordinate care for patients such as using your smartphone
- Respond appropriately to clinical decision-making supports and alerts
- Use information management tools to monitor outcomes of care processes

However, if the skillset you need is not yet developed, there are many opportunities today to develop these skills within your own practice. An important essential aspect is to understand the key computer hardware and software concepts and terminology and how these are all linked together to provide you with a better understanding of how computer and information literacy all tie to nursing informatics.

Software is defined as the applications and programs used by hardware to process information and data as discussed in Chapter 3—Hardware. Basically, hardware is the computer used for input, throughput, and output as defined in Chapter 3.

As you consider some of the experiences in your current practice using the EHR or other technology in general, do you understand all of the computer's functionality? Do you understand most of the terminology?

■ Question to Consider Before Reading On

1. *What is computer literacy? Why is it important to understand the concept?*

Computer Literacy and Concepts

Computer literacy today is broadly defined as having the skills, knowledge, and understanding to competently perform tasks using a computer. You may find different definitions if you search the Internet. You may also hear other terms such as "fluency" or "competencies" when referring to the ability to successfully and efficiently use a computer to complete a task.

In Chapter 3, the concept and description of computer hardware was introduced. In this chapter, you will continue to gain information regarding the many terms associated with computers, how to access different software applications, and the terminology. In this chapter, you will learn about essential computer software concepts and will have more discussion of different applications or "apps" and how to use them. Some of the references in this chapter are older but seminal, original, and substantial works that have not varied much in past years.

Questions to Consider Before Reading On

1. *What is software? What is the difference between hardware and software?*
2. *Define computer programs. List one function of a computer program.*
3. *What are data structures? What is the purpose of a data structure?*

What Is Software?

Computer software is that part of a computer system consisting of the computer programs and their associated data structures that direct the computer hardware to perform useful tasks desired by the user.

Computer Programs

A computer program is a list of instructions that tells the hardware the step-by-step operations to be performed to execute a task. It may gather input from the input devices, do calculations based on that input, make decisions based on those calculations, and store the results in the computer's memory, or send the results to output devices.

Computer programs are typically written in a *high-level language* that is similar to the designer's natural language and are translated by a utility program called a "compiler" into machine-level code that can be understood by the computer hardware.

Data Structures

The data structures associated with a computer program are the collection of information used by the program in accomplishing its tasks. This information may be of a more permanent form, such as lists of patients, their addresses, and so on, or it may be much more temporary such as the patient's current blood pressure or heart rate. The information is typically arranged in some type of database structure and is stored on the computer's secondary storage until it is brought into main memory for manipulation or modification.

■ Questions to Consider Before Reading On

1. *What is system software? What is included in system software?*
2. *Do you know which computer operating system (OS) you are using?*
3. *What are device drivers?*
4. *List one example of a utility program.*
5. *List one example of application software or "apps." What does the app you listed do—what is its function?*

■ Software Domains

Software generally falls into two general domains: system software and applications. System software works closely with the computer hardware and is made up of the OS and its device drivers and utility programs (see Figure 4.1).

Operating Systems

The concept of OSs was first introduced in Chapter 3. Starting with computer basics, defining the OSs and their functions is the first thing to consider as these are the first key steps to making a computer work. OSs are fundamental to making a computer work. They manage the computer's memory and processes, as well as all of its software and hardware. They also allow you to communicate with the computer without knowing how to speak the computer's language. Without an OS, only the simplest computers will work.

The OS usually comes already loaded on any computer you buy. Most people use the OS that comes with their computer, but it is possible to upgrade or even change OSs. The two most common OSs for personal computers are Microsoft Windows, which is used in over 80% of PCs worldwide, and Apple's MacOS, used in nearly 15% (see Desktop OSs at http://gs.statcounter.com/os-market-share/desktop/worldwide/#monthly-201711-2017 11-bar). Other OSs include Linux, which is a free and open source (freely available and not held under a restrictive copyright), used primarily in server and specialized applications, and Google Chrome OS. Chrome OS is used in Chromebooks, which are more basic and lower cost PCs used primarily for connection to the Internet (see Should I Buy a Chromebook? Buying Guide and Advice at www.laptopmag.com/articles/chromebook-buying-advice).

Personal devices such as smartphones and tablets use OSs that are different from, but related to, the OSs used in laptops and desktops. The iOS used in Apple smartphones and tablets is based on the same software as the MacOS used in the Apple desktop and laptop systems. The Android OS is widely used in non-Apple smartphones and tablets and has the largest installed base of any OS. Adaptations of Android are also used in cars, wrist watches, game consoles, cameras, and other smart devices (Goodwill Community Foundation, 2018).

Device Drivers

Device drivers are software contained within the OS that know the detail of how to interact with each of the hardware devices connected to the computer, such as hard drives, displays, keyboards, and Universal Serial Bus (USB) devices (defined in Chapter 3).

Utility Programs

Utility programs within the OS provide services to the computer users to maintain their hardware and software system. Examples would be Windows Backup and Restore and File History programs or MacOS's Time Machine program to copy or restore their system's hard drives to/from backup storage, or Display programs to control the computer's video display.

Application Software

Application software, or "apps" as it is more commonly known, is software that actually performs particular tasks needed by the user. It may be general purpose, such as word processing, building spreadsheets, or browsing the web, or it may be special purpose, such as managing EHRs. Examples of general purpose software include Microsoft Word for word processing or Microsoft Excel for spreadsheets. Web browsers include Microsoft's Internet Explorer, Mozilla's Firefox, Apple's Safari, Google's Chrome, and others.

General purpose software is frequently packaged in bundles, such as the Microsoft Office suite of programs, and web browsers are frequently packaged as part of the OS, as Microsoft's Internet Explorer is packaged with Microsoft Windows, and Apple's Safari is packaged with MacOS.

Examples of special purpose software would include photo management software such as Adobe Photoshop, personal finance software such as Quicken, or personal music management software such as iTunes. Special purpose software for EHR tasks includes Allscripts Professional EHR, Epic, or Cerner.

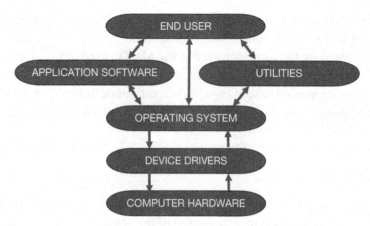

FIGURE 4.1 Categories of software and their relationships.

SOURCE: Sipes (2018).

Questions to Consider Before Reading On

1. *What is computer networking? Why is it important?*
2. *Define LAN. What is the purpose of LAN?*
3. *Define WAN. List two applications of WAN.*
4. *List one example of an IP address.*
5. *Define www. How is it used?*

Computer Networking

What Is Computer Networking?

Computer networking is the interconnection of two or more computer end-users to allow communication and resource sharing among the users. Users can communicate with each other using email or messaging applications, can share files with each other, and can share common equipment such as printers, scanners, and large disk storage.

Computer networking is generally described in terms of the physical scale of the network being used, that is, over how large a geographical area the users are distributed. Networks are categorized by the scope of their physical coverage; "Local Area Networks" (LANs) are typically limited in size to a home or building; geographically larger networks are termed "Wide Area Networks" (WANs) and are categorized by their size. Examples of computer networks and their applications are shown in Box 4.1 (Tanenbaum & Wetherall, 2010).

BOX 4.1

COMMON NETWORK TYPES AND APPLICATIONS

NETWORK TYPE	APPLICATION
Local Area Network	Home or business location
Campus Area Network	University or healthcare campus
Metropolitan Area Network	Citywide network; for example, multiple business locations
Wide Area Network	Intercity, continental, intercontinental locations
Internet	Worldwide network of networks

Local Area Networks

When computers are interconnected in a limited geographical area such as a home or a business location, they are interconnected by what is known as a LAN. The network may connect them using wireless technology known as Wi-Fi, or they may be interconnected by physical cables running through the walls using a wired technology called Ethernet.

Wi-Fi networks are more flexible to deploy, as users can easily be added to the network, but they can be susceptible to interference from things as mundane as microwave ovens and are potentially subject to "snooping" by outsiders. Ethernet cable networks are less flexible, as they require the physical connection of the computers to the cables, and the addition of new users may require running new cables through the walls. They are, however, less susceptible to interference and snooping.

Devices called "routers" are used to interconnect users on LANs. Routers "route" the traffic on the network between the right endpoints, as well as interconnect with the outside world, provide connection to network storage devices, and provide security functions such as firewall protection to the users on the LAN, as well as many other more complex technical functions (Figure 4.2).

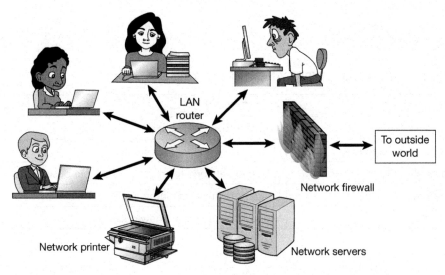

FIGURE 4.2 Local area network.

LAN, Local Area Network.

Wide Area Networks

When the distances between computer users become greater than what can be supported by LAN technology, it is necessary to use what are called WANs. The concepts of a WAN are not basically different from LANs, but the technology to accomplish the communication is different. The Wi-Fi or Ethernet technology used in LANs cannot transmit the network data over the tens or hundreds or thousands of miles needed to interconnect the users. The physical level technology used for WANs is much more akin to that used in long distance telephony, although the protocols used to manage and carry the data being transmitted are different. WANs are usually provided by telecommunications or cable companies as private networks that effectively are dedicated to the LANs that they interconnect, or on a shared basis as public networks (Figure 4.3).

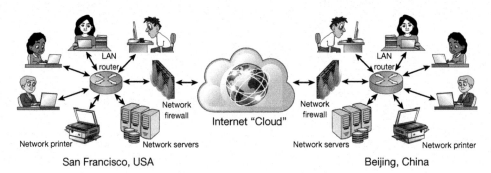

FIGURE 4.3 Wide area network using internet.

LAN, Local Area Network.

Internet

As more and more WANs were being used for commercial and academic purposes, the concept of interconnecting these networks into a network of networks emerged and became the Internet that exists today. These networks use a common method of communication, known as the "Internet protocol suite" (Transmission Control Protocol/Internet Protocol, or TCP/IP).

Every computer endpoint connected to the Internet is assigned an IP address and is connected through a router on its local LAN (or even directly) to a network access point provided by an Internet Service Provider (ISP). This connection is through a device known as a "modem" that adapts the technology used by the LAN to that used by the ISP, such as connection to the cable from a cable TV company, or to a telephone line for a telephone company's Digital Subscriber Line (DSL) service. The ISP provides services to the connected endpoints that may include network routing information, email service, and various security services, and connects them to a Network Service Provider (NSP) that provides the backbone transport service interconnected with other NSPs to form the Internet. The NSP does this through a network of very large, highly reliable routers that understand the topology of the Internet and will route the user's traffic to the terminating endpoint as efficiently as possible while avoiding points of severe congestion or failures (Perlman, 1999).

The scheme most widely used today for identifying endpoints on the Internet is IP Version 4 (IPv4), which was first introduced in 1983. IPv4 addresses are 32 bits in length, so that there are nearly 4.3 billion possible unique addresses. They are typically written in what is known as "dot-decimal notation," or as a series of four decimal numbers separated by periods, such as 117.182.0.1. As the Internet has grown, the number of available IPv4 addresses has been nearly exhausted, and a new addressing scheme known as IPv6 is being introduced. The new scheme uses a 128-bit address, which can provide as many as 3.4 with 38 zeros unique addresses. Although IPv4 and IPv6 are not interoperable, most network devices (routers, etc.) being marketed today are capable of working in either mode (see Box 4.2; Hinden & Deering, 2006).

BOX 4.2

IP ADDRESS FORM AND NOTATION

ADDRESS TYPE	ADDRESS SIZE	ADDRESS FORM	NUMBER OF POSSIBLE ADDRESSES
IPv4	32 bits	117.182.0.1	4.3 billion
IPv6	128 bits	ABCD:EF01:2345:6789: ABCD:EF01:2345:6789 Note: Hexadecimal (base 16) notation	3.4 with 38 zeros following

SOURCES: Socolofsky, T., & Kale, C. (1991).TCP/IP tutorial. RFC 1180. Retrieved from https://www.rfc-editor.org/info/rfc1180; Postel, J. (1982). Assigned numbers. RFC 820. Retrieved from https://www.rfc-editor.org/info/rfc820; Hinden, R., & Deering, S. (2006). IP Version 6 addressing architecture. RFC 4291. Retrieved from http://www.rfc-editor.org/info/rfc4291.

World Wide Web

The World Wide Web (also known as "the web") is a vast, worldwide information management system using hypertext links, or hyperlinks, embedded in documents to access other documents on the web. Documents and other resources on the web are addressed using a Uniform Resource Locator (URL) of the form www.google.com (Berners-Lee, Masinter, & McCahill, 1994). Access to the resources on the Web are over the Internet as the information transport vehicle.

Addresses on the web, as described by URLs, are divided into a number of "domains" to form a hierarchical addressing system. Box 4.3 lists the top-level domains in common use and their originally intended areas of application. Top-level domains have proliferated, and as of June, 2018, 1,543 top-level domains have been defined (see Daily TLD DNSSEC Report from ICANN Research at http://stats.research.icann.org/dns/tld_report).

Lower level domains are typically assigned on an organizational and functional basis and are separated in the domain name by periods. Subordinate pages within the domain are designated by "/" marks. As an example, https://ece.osu.edu/alumni/support/program is the website page for alumni to donate funds to the Electrical and Computer Engineering Department at The Ohio State University (Ohio State University Website, 2018).

BOX 4.3

COMMONLY USED TOP-LEVEL DOMAINS

TOP-LEVEL DOMAIN	ORIGINALLY INTENDED USE
.com	Commercial (now unrestricted)
.edu	Educational institution
.gov	U.S. federal government
.net	Network providers (now unrestricted)
.org	Nonprofit organizations (now unrestricted)
.mil	U.S. Armed Forces
.int	Certain international organizations

CASE SCENARIO

Josh is sharing information with colleagues at work discussing what he is learning in one of his nursing informatics courses in the nursing program at the local college. They begin to ask him questions about the differences between the Internet and World Wide Web and how each is used.

He does not remember all of the information he is just learning and is not sure where to go to find it. He begins a Google search by putting in key words such as "Internet," "World Wide Web," and finds much more information such as key features and uses of each. Based on this experience, he finds he can answer so many other questions as well as find directions on how to use each network more effectively and he begins to dig deeper into each explanation.

1. What are some searches Josh can complete? Where would he start to search for information about the Internet and World Wide Web?
2. He finds a document with an interesting explanation with ".com" in the title of the document. What does that mean? How important and relevant is the information in a .com document?
3. Is a .gov a better resource to answer his question?

▨ Questions to Consider Before Reading On

1. *Discuss how you would define web servers. What is the purpose of web servers?*
2. *What does HTML mean?*
3. *List three web browsers. Which one do you use?*

Resources on the web are provided on computer hardware and software systems known as "web servers" that are connected to the Internet. Collections of documents and resources on web servers are known as "websites" and consist of website pages. Web pages are typically written in a form of text known as Hypertext Markup Language (HTML), and communication between the end-user and the web server uses Hypertext Transfer Protocol (HTTP). End-users use application software called "web browsers" to access and display the information from the web. Examples of web browsers in use today are shown in Box 4.4.

BOX 4.4

POPULAR WEB BROWSERS

BROWSER NAME	PUBLISHER	REFERENCE
Edge (Formerly Internet Explorer)	Microsoft	https://www.microsoft.com/en-us/windows/microsoft-edge
Safari	Apple	https://www.apple.com/safari
Firefox	Mozilla	https://www.mozilla.org/en-US
Chrome	Google	https://www.google.com/chrome

Web pages do not always display correctly with all browsers due to differences in the features of different browsers. For this reason, it may be helpful to have multiple browsers loaded onto one's computer, so that if problems are encountered with accessing a web page with one browser, a different one can be tried.

Browsers have a number of settings that can be controlled by the user. For example, certain types of web pages called "pop-ups" can be blocked by the browser settings. While this can reduce the number of annoying ads that are displayed, it may also block useful information that a website is trying to display. For this reason, it is helpful to know how to change browser settings in case this problem arises. Similarly, since browsers typically store a historical list of websites visited and recent copies of websites displayed in a file called "cache," it is occasionally necessary to use the browser settings to "clear the cache" or history file to make a website work properly.

CASE SCENARIO (CONTINUED)

Josh has started his search to gain more information regarding the Internet and World Wide Web but now is having problems accessing the web page that was recommended as a good resource to use. He sees a notice on the page "Pop-Ups blocked." He ignores the message and tries to continue his Internet searches but finds he is unable to find what he wants.

He then begins to review what "Pop-Ups blocked" means, follows the directions he found for "allowing" pop-ups, then clears the pop-up by clicking on "allow pop-ups."

Questions:

1. What does pop-ups blocked mean?
2. What does "allowing" pop-ups do when trying to conduct Internet searches?
3. How can he determine which browser he is using?
4. What can he do to resolve this issue?

Browsers also store data sent by a website called "cookies" so that the website can keep track of the interaction with the users. Cookies can identify information about whether the user has logged in to the site and hence should have access to certain information, about purchases that have been loaded into a cart for an online purchase, whether the user has visited the site previously and has configured certain aspects of the site such as the user's name, and to what information the user should have access.

QSEN SCENARIO

You are working with a colleague who recognizes you are taking nursing informatics courses and learning about computer software. She asks you what topics you are covering, then asks what this has to do with your improving clinical practice. How would you respond?

▨ Questions to Consider Before Reading On

1. *List three of the most common search engines.*
2. *How are search engines used in clinical practice? In nursing college programs?*
3. *What is cloud computing? Discuss applications of cloud computing.*
4. *Define IoT. What are some of the future projects and applications coming out of IoT?*

■ Applications of the Internet and the World Wide Web

Search

One of the most useful applications of the Internet and the web is finding information to answer a question or to solve a problem. But there are nearly 1.9 billion websites (see Internet Live Stats, www.internetlivestats.com/watch/websites) on the Internet. So how is one to find the answers one needs?

In the earliest days of the web, information about websites was compiled and lists maintained by hand. In 1992, the list contained the addresses of 30 servers worldwide for information retrieval (www.w3.org/History/19921103-hypertext/hypertext/DataSources/WWW/Servers.html). As the web continued to grow rapidly, search engines, or automated tools for cataloging information on the web and making it accessible to regular users, were developed. Today there are literally hundreds of different search engines available, many of which are tailored to particular types of searches. Box 4.5 lists some of the most popular search engines in use today.

BOX 4.5

POPULAR SEARCH ENGINES

SEARCH ENGINE	REFERENCE	COMMENT
Google Search	https://www.google.com	Largest market share
Bing Search	https://www.bing.com	Microsoft's entry in Search
DuckDuckGo	https://duckduckgo.com	Does not collect your personal information
Yahoo Search	https://www.yahoo.com	Part of web portal
Webopedia	https://www.webopedia.com	Dictionary of technical terms

---

Cloud Computing

According to the National Institute of Standards and Technology's official definition, "Cloud computing is a model for enabling ubiquitous, convenient, on-demand network access to a shared pool of configurable computing resources (e.g., networks, servers, storage, applications and services) that can be rapidly provisioned and released with minimal management effort or service provider interaction" (Mell & Grance, 2011, p. 2).

To the user this means that applications and data are available that do not reside on his or her computer or local server, but rather on shared online servers that are accessed through the Internet "cloud." Computing resources, storage, and applications are available on a virtual or shared basis and are available from any device that has access to the Internet. Many cloud services are accessed through browser software, making them agnostic to computer type. Others may be accessed through special "client" software loaded on the user's computer, but usually available for various computers and OSs. Box 4.6 lists several general purpose cloud services that can be used to store files to be shared with others, for backup storage for the user's computer system, or general purpose applications.

BOX 4.6

GENERAL PURPOSE CLOUD SERVICES

GENERAL PURPOSE CLOUD SERVICES	APPLICATION	REFERENCE
iCloud	Storage, backup, email, productivity suite	https://www.apple.com/icloud
Google Drive	Storage, backup, file sharing	https://www.google.com/drive
Microsoft OneDrive	Storage, backup, file sharing	https://onedrive.live.com/about/en-us
Google Docs	Word processing	https://www.google.com/docs/about
Google Sheets	Spreadsheets	https://www.google.com/sheets/about
Google Slides	Presentations	https://www.google.com/slides/about
Microsoft Office 365	Office productivity suite	https://products.office.com/en-US/?ms.url=office365com
Amazon Web Services	Hosting platform for business services	https://aws.amazon.com/what-is-aws

---

Many special purpose applications are also cloud based today, including many in the EHR/electronic medical record field. Cloud-based EHR systems can offer healthcare providers significant benefits, in that the clinical data are shared in the cloud and not limited to users who are in the same location as the software and servers. Examples of cloud-based healthcare applications are shown in Box 4.7.

BOX 4.7

SOME SPECIAL PURPOSE CLOUD SERVICES

SPECIAL PURPOSE CLOUD SERVICE	APPLICATION	REFERENCE
AthenaHealth	EHR	https://www.athenahealth.com
AllegianceMD	EHR	https://allegiancemd.com
AllScripts	EHR	https://www.allscripts.com

Internet of Things

The Internet of Things (IoT) is the network of "smart" devices that are connected to the Internet and have embedded software and sensors that enable them to interoperate without requiring human interaction. Many have basic learning capabilities, allowing them to learn and adapt to their input data and adjust their output behavior accordingly.

Examples of "Things" in the IoT sense include smart thermostats and smart light bulbs that automatically adjust temperature or lighting based on the user's habits, and wearable devices to monitor various physical indicators such as pulse rate and blood pressure.

The healthcare field offers many opportunities for the application of IoT. A company named Qardio is developing a family of "connected" devices to remotely monitor a patient's vital signs, including a wearable ECG claimed to track complete heart health on his or her smartphone and share the data with his or her doctor automatically (see www .getqardio.com/qardiocore-wearable-ecg-ekg-monitor-iphone).

Zanthion, a start-up company in San Francisco, is focusing on a Senior Care Platform comprising a suite of integrated wearable devices and environmental sensors that provide a complete view of an elderly patient's daily life to alert to the need for intervention or emergency support (see www.zanthion.com).

The National Health Service (NHS) in the UK has been conducting a Test Bed program (a group of 40 innovators, 51 digital products, and five voluntary sector organizations) of NHS–Innovator partnerships to evaluate the introduction of integrated digital technology and IoT into the healthcare system to improve patient outcomes at equivalent or lower cost than current practice. The program is currently concluding its initial evaluation of the first seven Test Beds, several of which focused on the use of connected IoT devices for monitoring and management of conditions such as chronic obstructive pulmonary disease (COPD), diabetes, heart failure, and mild-to-moderate dementia. Devices used included wearables to monitor patients' vital signs as well as Global Positioning System (GPS) trackers, door and electricity monitors, and motion sensors. A second wave of Test Beds focusing on type 2 diabetes and several other priority areas is currently in the planning stage (Galea, Hough, & Khan, 2017).

Questions to Consider Before Reading On

1. *Why is understanding computer security important?*
2. *Define malware. Discuss different forms of malware. What can happen if there is a malware "attack?"*
3. *List three steps to prevent malware attacks.*

Computer Security

Malware is software developed to damage or otherwise gain unapproved access to computers without official approval. Anything that is connected to the Internet can be disrupted, damaged, or subject to unauthorized access. Malware has been around for nearly as long as the Internet. In recent years, as the world has become more and more interconnected and dependent on the Internet, a recent report by the U.S. President's Council of Economic Advisors (CEA) estimated that cybercrime cost the U.S. economy between $57 billion and $109 billion in 2016 (https://www.whitehouse.gov/wp-content/uploads/2018/03/The-Cost-of-Malicious-Cyber-Activity-to-the-U.S.-Economy.pdf). In May, 2017, a worldwide cyberattack by the malware variant was Wanna Decryptor; "cryptoworm" crippled parts of the National Health System (NHS) in the UK, disrupting services at one-third of the hospital trusts in England and infecting a further 603 primary care and physicians' facilities with demands for ransom (www.england.nhs.uk/wp-content/uploads/2018/02/lessons-learned-review-wannacry-ransomware-cyber-attack-cio-review.pdf).

Malware can come in a number of different forms, known as "viruses," "bacterium," "worms," and "Trojan horses," depending on how they behave and are spread. Their effects can destroy computer files or launch coordinated attacks on websites as botnets. Ransomware can encrypt user files on infected computers with demands for payment to decrypt the files.

There are some basic steps that the end-user can take to prevent or reduce the probability of infection by malware (see Box 4.8). Some of these will be implemented by IT in a corporate environment, but others are dependent on the behavior of individuals.

BOX 4.8

WAYS TO PREVENT MALWARE ATTACKS

- Use firewalls—Firewalls are hardware or software designed to prevent unauthorized intrusion. Most routers include firewall protection, and corporate networks will certainly include them.
- Use antivirus software—Antivirus software will scan the computer's files and identify and quarantine malware that it finds. Many also scan files being downloaded from websites.

(continued)

BOX 4.8 (*continued*)

- Use encryption—When accessing websites, look for https rather than http in the URL together with the padlock emoji 🔒 to indicate that your browser is encrypting the information being exchanged with the website.

- Stay current on software updates—The WannaCry ransomware attack in May 2017 was focused on a vulnerability in Microsoft Windows that had been identified, and a patch to prevent such an attack had been released by Microsoft in March 2017.

- Use strong passwords or password managers—Strong, hard to guess passwords that are not shared with coworkers are a key defense. Password managers such as 1Password (https://1password.com), LastPass (www.lastpass.com), or Dashlane (www.dashlane.com) are alternatives for creating and managing strong passwords. And do not reuse passwords for multiple websites; if the password is broken for one site, it is easily broken for all of them.

- Do not open email attachments that you are not expecting—Email attachments are the way many malware infections occur. Just because you recognize the name of the sender does not make it safe, as many cybercriminals know how to "spoof" the sender's name.

- Do not click on web links in email messages—As with email attachments, clicking on web links in email messages will frequently cause malware downloads to your computer. Again, just because you recognize the name of the sender does not make it safe, as many cybercriminals know how to "spoof" the sender's name.

- Do not load software or data from unknown memory sticks—Connecting USB memory sticks (flash drives, thumb drives) from unknown sources or with unknown contents is a good way to become infected. Many corporate networks disable the USB ports or forbid employees from using personal USB memory sticks to prevent such infections.

Following a few basic rules as outlined in Box 4.8, both in the personal and in the professional healthcare environment, will go a long way toward maintaining a safe Internet environment (see Transunion, www.transunion.com/blog/identity-protection/why-is-cyber-security-important; Kaufman, Perlman, & Speciner, 2002).

■ Critical Thinking Questions and Activities

- *Identify the OS you are currently using. How and where did you find this information on your computer?*

- *In Box 4.6, there is a list of cloud computing services and applications. Which one(s) are you using? What is the application you are using it for?*

- *You find a flash drive lying on your desk and believe it is the one you just discussed with a friend. What are some things you need to check before loading it onto your computer?*

- *You receive an email from another school with a link included in the message. It instructs you to open the link to see a message from a friend. You do not know anyone at that school. What should you do?*

- *In a message subject line the tile is "Unclaimed money can be yours." You open the message which states a large amount of money has been found with your name. You just need to send your bank ID numbers, address, phone number, and where you currently work. What would you do in this case?*

- *Discuss how computers are used by nurses in different healthcare settings, that is, acute care, home health, school nursing, and others you might think of.*

SUMMARY

This chapter provides important information regarding the software applications frequently used. Examples of the different software types for managing information were included. System software works closely with the computer hardware and is made up of the OS and two main programs—device drivers and utility programs.

Computer networking, the interconnection of two or more computer end-users, was discussed, with examples of LAN and WAN systems needed for communication and resource sharing among the users. Discussion and definitions of the Internet and World Wide Web were included with an example application in the case scenario.

More recently, there is information on cloud computing and how it can benefit users. Examples and applications were provided as well as information on different types and uses of browsers, including a case scenario on pop-up blockers.

The very important section on computer security included examples of malware attacks and consequences to industry. It included ways to prevent malware attacks in addition to critical thinking questions and activities to engage the reader as well as reinforce important concepts.

References

Berners-Lee, T., Masinter, L., & McCahill, M. (1994). Uniform resource locators (URL). Retrieved from https://www.rfc-editor.org/info/rfc1738

Casey, H. (2018). Should I buy a Chromebook? Buying guide and advice. Retrieved from https://www.laptopmag.com/articles/chromebook-buying-advice

Council of Economic Advisors. (2016). The cost of malicious cyber activity to the U.S. economy. Retrieved from https://www.whitehouse.gov/wp-content/uploads/2018/03/The-Cost-of-Malicious-Cyber-Activity-to-the-U.S.-Economy.pdf

Cronenwett, L., Sherwood, G., Pohl, J., Barnsteiner, J., Moore, S., Sullivan, D. T., . . . & Warren, J. (2009). Quality and safety education for advanced nursing practice. *Nursing Outlook, 57*(6), 338–348. doi: 10.1016/j.outlook.2009.07.009.

Galea, A., Hough, E., & Khan, I. (2017). *Test beds—The story so far*. England, London: National Health System. Retrieved from https://www.england.nhs.uk/ourwork/innovation/test-beds

Goodwill Community Foundation. (2018). Computer basics: Understanding operating systems. Retrieved from https://www.gcflearnfree.org/computerbasics/understanding-operating-systems

Hinden, R., & Deering, S. (2006). IP Version 6 addressing architecture. RFC 4291. Retrieved from http://www.rfc-editor.org/info/rfc4291

ICANN Research. (2018). Daily TLD DNSSEC Report. Retrieved from http://stats.research .icann.org/dns/tld_report

Internet Live Stats. (2018). Websites. Retrieved from http://www.internetlivestats.com/watch/ websites

Kaufman, C., Perlman, R., & Speciner, M. (2002). *Network security: Private communication in a public world* (2nd ed.). Upper Saddle River, NJ: PTR Prentice Hall.

Mell, P., & Grance, T. (2011). *The NIST definition of cloud computing (technical report).* National Institute of Standards and Technology: U.S. Department of Commerce. Special publication 800-145. Retrieved from https://nvlpubs.nist.gov/nistpubs/legacy/sp/ nistspecialpublication800-145.pdf

Ohio State University Website. (2018). Electrical and computer engineering (ECE) department https://ece.osu.edu/alumni/support/program

Perlman, R. (1999). *Interconnections: Bridges, routers, switches, and internetworking protocols* (2nd ed.). Addison-Wesley Professional Computing Series. Boston, MA: Addison Wesley.

Postel, J. (1982). Assigned numbers. RFC 820. Retrieved from https://www.rfc-editor.org/ info/rfc820

Socolofsky, T., & Kale, C. (1991). TCP/IP tutorial. RFC 1180. Retrieved from https://www .rfc-editor.org/info/rfc1180

Statcounter. (2018). Desktop operating systems. Retrieved from http://gs.statcounter.com/ os-market-share/desktop/worldwide/#monthly-201711-201711-bar

Tanenbaum, A. S., & Wetherall, D. (2010). *Computer networks.* Upper Saddle River, NJ: Pearson Prentice Hall.

Transunion. (2017). Why is cyber security important? Identify protection. Retrieved from https://www.transunion.com/blog/identity-protection/why-is-cyber-security-important

PART III

NURSING INFORMATICS: CLINICAL APPLICATIONS

CHAPTER 5

NURSING INFORMATICS: PROJECT MANAGEMENT

CAROLYN SIPES

LEARNING OBJECTIVES AND OUTCOMES

Upon completion of this chapter, the reader will be able to:

- Discuss the correlation among nursing informatics, nursing process, project management and systems development life cycle (SDLC).
- Discuss Health Information Technology for Economic and Clinical Health (HITECH), its implications for your practice, and why it is important.
- Discuss the meaningful-use initiative and why it is important.
- Discuss how it has impacted your practice.

⊙ KEY NURSING INFORMATICS TERMS

Some of the key concepts and terms you will hear in the practice and discipline of nursing informatics are:

Acceptance testing	Execution
American Recovery and Reinvestment Act (ARRA)	Health Information Technology for Economic and Clinical Health (HITECH)
Clinical workflows	Implementation
Closing	Information literacy
Computer literacy	Initiation
Electronic health records (EHRs)	Lessons learned
End user/Super-users	Meaningful use

⊙ **KEY NURSING INFORMATICS TERMS** (*continued*)

Nursing informatics standards of practice

Nursing process

Planning

Project management life cycle (PLC)

Systems development life cycle (SDLC)

Testing

Usability

Workflows

Work breakdown structure (WBS)

INTRODUCTION: PROJECT MANAGEMENT

Consider what you already know about the roles of an informatics nurse (IN), including nursing informatics (NI) skills and competencies, understanding the nursing process and how it correlates with the PLC, and SDLC. You ask, Why do I need to know this and how will knowing this apply to my role as a nurse and my clinical practice? These questions and more are discussed in this chapter.

You may have been involved in explaining your current workflow and what is needed in the new system, creating the new workflows, providing recommendations for how you complete your daily tasks caring for patients. This would be done using the new EHR clinical system after implementation, during which you had to learn new documentation skills to record patient information in the computer. You may have had to learn new terminology such as *end user* or *clinical workflows*. How do you think understanding clinical workflows impacted your practice, if at all?

This chapter focuses on understanding the value and skills nurses need to develop when learning the principles of project management and how these correlate with what you already know through application of the nursing process. Understanding project management concepts takes this process a step further by providing guidelines for what the healthcare information system is and how it works.

In addition, this chapter identifies many of the new trends and roles nurses are involved in when an organization decides to buy and implement a new clinical computer system. Because nurses comprise the largest discipline using EHRs, they are asked to help provide recommendations and feedback in every aspect of their design, planning and implementation, and to then evaluate what works and what needs to be corrected when a new clinical system is purchased by the healthcare facility.

▓ Questions to Consider Before Reading on

1. *What is project management and the PLC? How is it different from SDLC?*

2. *Why is it important to understand the processes of project management?*

3. *How do you think understanding project management might apply to your practice? What are some of the skills an IN might use in project management?*

4. *List three phases of PLC. Discuss the tasks you have identified for each phase.*

5. *What are the critical questions to ask before any project is approved? Were nurses involved in helping to facilitate understanding of their workflow?*

What Is Project Management?

For many, the idea of doing project management is daunting. But understating the basic concepts of project management, the PLC, and how and where to apply them can be simple regardless of the size or purpose of the project. Just as you used a standardized process with your first patient assessments, project managers also use a standardized process.

Using consistent, standard processes in an organized way helps to meet any project goals and objectives. For example, for a project, such as an EHR implementation, all aspects must be expertly managed to deliver the on-time, on-budget outcomes.

Of the NI competencies and roles discussed in Chapter 2, project management is one of the most important item identified as it impacts all areas of NI skills and provides an organizing framework for nursing processes and projects, including having the skill to understand what happens in each phase, such as design, planning, implementation, follow-up, and evaluation. Project management, then, is the application of knowledge, skills, tools, and techniques to project activities so as to meet the project requirements, such as the activities involved with implementing a new clinical EHR.

Other examples of job roles that specifically require project management skills as an essential part of NI functions include management, administration, leadership, faculty, graduate-level master's and doctorate practicum courses. But first, a better understanding of the skills essential to NI, including those of project management, is vital before adequate education and training programs can be developed (Sipes, 2016a, b).

As previously discussed, the standard processes used by INs and project managers are very similar to the steps followed in the nursing process. They include a list of activities or tasks that need to be completed during each phase of a project before the next step can be started. In very general terms, the Project Management Institute's (PMI) *A Guide to the Project Management Body of Knowledge* (PMBOK® Guide, 2017) defines the five major phases and processes of project management. Similar to the NI standards of practice, these are:

- Design/initiation
- Planning
- Execution/implementation
- Monitoring and control
- Closing/evaluation and lessons learned

An overview of the tasks included in each phase is provided in Box 5.1.

Differences Between Project Management Life Cycle and Systems Development Life Cycle

For project management, the Project Life Cycle (PLC) focuses on the phases, processes, tools, knowledge, and skills needed to manage a project. *Project management* is defined as the management of a project from start to finish. It requires excellent communication, knowledge, and organizational skills to manage the five phases listed as well as team building (Project Management Institute [PMI], 2017). The PLC is a process project managers are responsible for and use to develop and "go-live or bring up" the new EHR, for example, including not only the clinical system but administrative components that include patient demographic data for billing.

The System Development Life Cycle (SDLC) you may hear about is not the same and only a subpart of the PLC, used for developing particular software products needed for the larger project or may be part of solving a specific software problem, more information technology (IT) focused (Cunningham, 2018).

Further, the definition of a project is that it is something unique, not a routine operation done every day, but a specific set of operations designed to accomplish a singular goal such as design and implementation of a new EHR. A project team often includes people who usually do not work together—sometimes they come from different organizations and across multiple geographies, depending on the skill set needed for the project.

In contrast to the nursing process (see Box 5.1), these five project management processes are the ones most frequently used. However, larger projects may break down the processes into six or more components, or phases, so that the project can more easily be controlled; some smaller organizations only use four—this all depends on the organization. Regardless, the tasks identified in each phase must be completed before moving on—just as you would when applying the nursing process. Would you implement a care plan without first completing the assessment of your patient?

BOX 5.1

CORRELATION AMONG NURSING INFORMATICS STANDARDS, NURSING PROCESS, AND PROJECT MANAGEMENT

NURSING INFORMATICS STANDARDS	NURSING PROCESS	PROJECT MANAGEMENT
Std: 1. Assessment—the IN collects data and information	1. Assessment—collect and analyze patient data	1. Design/Initiate project—current state workflow analysis; gap analysis; scope, charter
Std 4. Planning—the IN develops a plan	2. Diagnosis; develop precare plan	2. Plan/develop project plan
Std. 5: Implementation—the IN implements plan	3. Outcomes plan; goal development	3. Execute/implement project plan; go-live
Std. 5a: Coordination—the IN coordinates activities	4. Implement care plan	4. Monitor and control project risk management;change control

(continued)

BOX 5.1 *(continued)*

NURSING INFORMATICS STANDARDS	NURSING PROCESS	PROJECT MANAGEMENT
Std. 6: Evaluation—the IN evaluates attainment of outcomes	5. Evaluate plan; update plan	5. Close project; evaluate lessons learned
Final assessments—Overall assessment: Will it improve patient quality and safety?		

IN, informatics nurse.

SOURCE: Adapted from Sipes (2016a, b).

Project management requires managing a process from start to finish using excellent communication skills and the ability to organize and complete tasks following the five phases listed in Box 5.1. Organizing the project following specific steps adds a structure and a framework that makes it much easier to track, change, or modify as needed before moving to the next phase.

Basic principles and an increased understanding of project management are frequently acquired over a number of projects; learning what works well and where to focus key time and resources takes time and experience, especially after lessons learned from previous projects have been evaluated. Just as you provide the care plan for your patient, the second time you assess for the same diagnosis it becomes a bit easier with experience. Just as in clinical practice, there are questions to ask first during a critical analysis before the design and final approval project of the project and includes:

▶ **Questions to Ask Before Any Project Is Approved**

- Why are we doing this project? (Is it to replace an old system?)
- Why do we need it? Who will benefit?
- How will it impact my practice?
- Will it improve patient quality and safety?

Whatever the decision is regarding the need for a new EHR, it is important to set clear expectations for all involved at all levels of patient care indicating what is needed so all participants have some understanding of what the new system can and should provide. Nurses are asked to provide requirements for their daily work requirements, new workflow diagrams should be developed for the new system and gaps in the flow of current patient care tasks are identified so they can be addressed and the correct flow built into the new system. This provides a process so that patient care is provided in an organized way (See Figure 5.3).

■ Questions to Consider Before Reading on

1. *Why is it important to understand correlations between the nursing process and project management process? How do each of these compare to the other in terms of the different tasks that have to be completed in each phase?*

2. *How should nurses be involved when a new EHR system is implemented in their healthcare facility?*

3. *How will a new EHR potentially impact current, daily practice? What are the pros and cons of a new system?*

■ Newer Trends in Nursing Practice Roles

With the advent of the American Recovery and Reinvestment Act (ARRA), which contained the Health Information Technology for Economic and Clinical Health Act (HITECH Act), came the mandate of what healthcare workers "should do, including using EHRs to collect and monitor patient data, which further encouraged the use and development of technology by all nurses" (HITECH Act, 2009, p. 1). The Act's accompanying funding resources stimulated more rapid movement toward electronic data capture and health information exchanges (HIE; American Recovery and Reinvestment Act [ARRA], 2009).

Historically, President George W. Bush outlined a plan to ensure that most Americans have an EHR by 2014, and stated that "by computerizing health records we can avoid dangerous medical mistakes, reduce costs, and improve care" (President George W. Bush, State of the Union Address, January 20, 2004, p. 1). Then, in 2009, the HITECH Act, enacted as part of the ARRA of 2009, developed incentives for providers to demonstrate "meaningful use" of EHRs (ARRA, 2014) by changing from paper systems or changing older system to those now certified based on government regulations. To be competent as an EHR user requires competencies in informatics, specifically, data entry, analysis, facilitation between IT and clinicians, workflow design, and change management (HealthIT Policy, 2014).

However, a key factor was overlooked when this mandate was presented; there are very few people in the workforce who are competent or possess the skills needed to implement any of the recommendations without extensive training. Many of the skills needed to undertake any role, large or small, to stay well organized and managed, include:

■ Good communication skills and processes—both verbal and written

■ Understanding the steps in the planning and implementation processes that also require close monitoring, just as you with a patient's condition, it is the same with any project, such as EHR development

■ Monitoring for potential risks and need for or use of resources

■ Controlling quality through a variety of processes

■ Evaluating and mitigating problems

This list requires a skill mix of computer and information literacy as well as NI at all levels of practice, especially when computer literacy is defined as more technical and involves knowledge of how to use a computer. *Information literacy* is defined as the ability to find and evaluate sources of information with careful consideration of all information sources to be used; not a simple task. For example, there may be many sources of information, but not all of them are reliable or trustworthy. Learning to recognize which sources are relevant to the issue—using critical thinking to make clinical decisions that will affect someone's life—"is a crucial skill for nurses and other healthcare professionals to develop" (American Library Association [ALA], 2014, p. 1). Can you imagine how tracking any of these roles and skills would be done without the use of a computer or other technology?

With the recommendations of the ARRA and this accompanying mandate that hospitals implement EHRs, there is an even greater need to implement a standardized, organizing process and methodology to effectively and efficiently guide organizations through the many tasks needed to implement especially complex EHRs in a very systematic way. Project management provides these standard processes, just as the NI standards of practice and the nursing process provide a step-wise, organized process for the provision of patient care.

Today, the concept of project management has become a key management strategy in large corporations, such as IBM, Apple, Microsoft and other industries, required through the Meaningful Use (MU) initiative where hospitals have to demonstrate they are using EHRs in a meaningful way. In health care at all levels where there is a need to put a formalized structure and organization to tasks carried out in organizations.

As discussed above, learning the principles of project management are very similar concepts to the nursing process. Not only are the steps that are used to manage patient care required in practice, all nurses are expected to possess the skills and ability to apply concepts of project management now more than eve practice.

The American Nurses Association (ANA; 2015) and the Healthcare Information Management Systems Society (HIMSS; 2014; Sipes et al., 2016) emphasize that "informatics competencies are needed by **all** nurses whether or not they specialize in informatics. As nurse settings become more ubiquitous computing environments, all nurses must be both information and computer literate" (p. 1). As discussed in Chapter 2, the ANA's (2008) *Nursing Informatics: Scope and Standards of Practice* identify methodologies and technology used in informatics as part of project management in that the knowledge, techniques, and competencies required and developed by using NI help nurses better manage their practice.

Although the concept of project management seems foreign to many, there is a common thread that applies to the different types of work that nurses do (i.e., the nursing process—one of the first core principles of nursing practice that nurses learn to use when delivering the best evidence-based patient care). The suggestion that nurses will understand and be able to apply the five phases of project management arises from project management's similarity to the five steps of the nursing process. The terminology for some of the steps and phases is similar among the three processes but the differences may be only an issue of semantics. The main differences are that they are working with a project instead of patients.

Figures 5.1 and 5.2 include the five steps of the nursing process and the five-step project management processes.

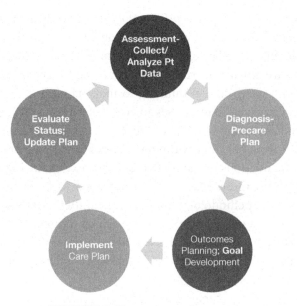

FIGURE 5.1 Five-step nursing process.

Pt, patient.

SOURCE: Sipes (2016a).

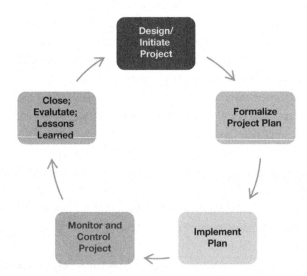

FIGURE 5.2 Five-step process used for project management and SDLC.

SDLC, systems development life cycle.

SOURCE: Sipes (2016a, b).

▧ Questions to Consider Before Reading on

1. *Discuss why it is important to understand the different tasks in each phase of project management.*

2. *How will understanding an organizing framework help add structure to any process you might use?*

3. *Discuss the five phases of project management. How do they correlate with the nursing process and standards of practice for NI?*

4. *Discuss how developing a workflow of something you might want to do, such as planning an event at work, would be beneficial.*

▨ Phases of Project Management

The five phases of project management were briefly outlined previously. This section outlines and provides information regarding the different tasks that are completed in the various phases. The SDLC, as defined above, is a sub phase of project management were the focus is on the development of only one application or component of a whole project and has phases within the sub phase, so will not be discussed further. The main focus is on the five phases of the larger project management concepts.

Phase 1: Design/Initiation

The first step when launching any project is to conduct and analyze what is known as the *current state. Current state* refers to reviewing the "what is"—what is currently happening and then looking to define what and/or where the gaps might be—what is missing or what could be done better in a workflow. For example, one of the reasons a project might have been proposed is the need for a remodel, an upgrade, to solve some problem, such as long patient wait times, or to add something new that would expedite a process, for example, improving the clinical documentation or medication-ordering processes. Overall, the project is being implemented to meet a need, and the need or gap should be justified with documentation of workflows that indicate any gaps.

When beginning to diagram a workflow, the first step is to start by drawing boxes that will represent each step in the process until arriving at a step where there is a gap in the flow–the gap analysis (Figure 5.3)–the gaps in the process should be clearly evident.

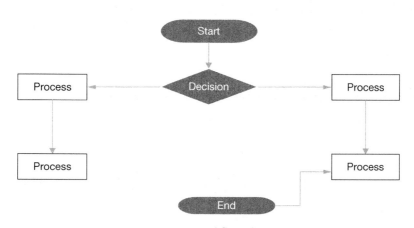

FIGURE 5.3 Workflow diagram.

SOURCE: Sipes (2018).

It is important to do this first by just sketching the diagram quickly on a note pad while working with others who may be providing information so that thought processes are not lost. As frequently happens, the process will include a review and may be revised a number of times. As end users start to think through the processes, with repeated review they will begin to remember more details, especially if they are working with others to document the workflow. After several iterations have been completed, the diagram can be formally documented, especially if using a program called *Microsoft Visio*. If one is not familiar with this program, there may be a steep learning curve to learn how to use it, but there may be no time to do so. Many times, organizations have someone on the project who has experience using the application.

CASE SCENARIO

Camille has just learned the hospital where she works is deciding on a vendor to use when they purchase and implement a new clinical information system (EHR) next year. She is very concerned about what this means as many of her coworkers state they will not be happy with the new system because they will have to learn more computer skills that will take more time away from patient care. They have heard many stories from others who have just gone through this experience and found it very disruptive to daily workflows. Some nurses from neighboring hospitals left due to the turmoil.

Camille's coworkers have expressed concerns and are wondering why all of these changes are needed when everything is "working fine." They are not in favor of this change.

When considering questions to ask, Camille starts to explore the benefits of a new EHR. Questions she asks include:

1. How will the new system be implemented?
2. What roles will nurses have to play in the design, planning, and implementation of the new system?
3. Will there be training to use the new system?
4. How long will it all take?
5. What are some of the benefits of the new system that will improve my clinical workflows?

▦ Questions to Consider Before Reading on

1. *What does setting goals entail?*
2. *Why is it important to set goals and review expectations?*
3. *Discuss one way to set a goal so that it can be measured.*

Setting Project Goals and Expectations

Critical to the detail is the inclusion of measurable, well-defined goals and objectives. A *goal* is defined as a general statement about some task or project that needs to be accomplished. The objectives define the steps that determine how the goal(s) will be accomplished and help keep the project moving. How are the five Ws and H (who, what, when, where, why, and how) used to develop measurable objectives? Why do you think it is important to be able to measure and evaluate objectives?

Many find it difficult to develop well-defined, specific goals and objectives, leading to adequately tracking whether the missing item has been completed. Well-defined goals and objectives include details and metrics such as:

Number of units involved—How many?

Specific tasks to be completed—How many, which ones, and when are they due?

What are due dates for all tasks and subtasks?

Who is the owner? Is this person different from those who have final responsibility?

Writing SMART Objectives

The plan objectives should be developed as SMART objectives, meaning they need to be _s_pecific, _m_easurable, _a_chievable (attainable), _r_elevant, and _t_imely. The key to developing critical, measurable objectives is to have collectable data that are adequate for measuring change. You can think of a well-defined objective by answering the five Ws and H questions of who, what, where, when, why and how. You also need to detail "how" the tasks will be accomplished (Box 5.2; Nightingale College, 2016).

BOX 5.2

THE FIVE Ws AND H OF MEASURABLE OBJECTIVES; WRITING SMART OBJECTIVES

When writing SMART measureable objectives—use the five Ws and H (Sipes, 2016a)—the "who, what, when, where, why, and how" to help define measureable metrics.

Who and what department or role needs to perform the activities?
Who will the project impact?
Who will pay for the project?
Who is making the decisions?
What are the benefits and to whom do they apply?
Where will this occur?
When will the different activities be completed?
Why is this project being done?
How will this be completed? Is there a list of tasks and resources (Sipes, 2016a)?

Defining Scope and Charter

The next big task is to define the scope and charter which defined many of the key elements of the project. The scope document is a formal document that details how the project will be managed and what the project requirements are. It defines the boundaries of what can and cannot be done.

After the scope document is approved by the key stakeholders, any additional or further change will need to go through the change management process and be approved by stakeholders and other key leadership. The scope document should address the problem or opportunity that will be resolved with the implementation of the project. It defines the project goal and objectives and the metrics that will be used to determine the success of the project. In this phase of design, a number of key project management documents are created, including the charter, which adds the framework for the "who, what, when, why, where, and how," so the project can proceed (Sipes, 2016a). The project charter is based on the outcomes of the workflow/gap analysis and defines the roles and responsibilities of the project team members, outlines the project objectives, identifies the main stakeholders, defines the authority of the project manager, and authorizes the project with formal sign-off.

A needs assessment, also referred to as the *workflow gap analysis*, includes a review of the current state of the project (see Figure 5.3) as well as its anticipated future state information. The workflow analysis helps to define and organize basic draft ideas into a more comprehensive format that is easier to follow. The needs assessment contains the evaluation of the business need for the project as well as the anticipated outcome of the project.

Questions to Consider Before Reading on

1. *Discuss the value of a developing a work breakdown structure (WBS).*
2. *How can this type of structure impact and help organize practice?*

Phase 2: Planning

After the design/initiation phase of project management is completed, it is time to begin the planning phase of the project. This phase is one of the most important phases of the project. If tasks or activities are not identified and planned during this phase, it can cause delays in the overall project. A detailed, very specific project plan is key to setting the expectations for the five "Ws" and an "H": the who, what, when, where, why, and how of a project (Sipes, 2016a), described previously. All of these specific details will have been outlined in the project objectives during the design phase, and now can now be revised and updated.

Steps in Project Planning

Planning in project management is like a road map that gives the detail necessary for the project to navigate the project highway and finish successfully. Many of the project requirements build on one another and can be revised and updated as more details of the project are defined and monitored through a change management plan. Many of the tools and different variations of tools can be found on the web.

The planning phase builds on the processes established in the design phase and develops the work breakdown structure (WBS) and schedules using the defined steps of project planning, which include:

1. Build a project scope based on the project charter.
2. Break down the scope into tasks/work packages.
3. Assign tasks/work packages to their owners.
4. Task/work package owners build activity lists.
5. Activity owners estimate or calculate activity durations.
6. As a team, activity owners sequence activities.
7. Identify and document dependencies.
8. Build a schedule based on these steps.

The example of one format used to help see what needs to be done in a much easier way is presented in Figure 5.4.

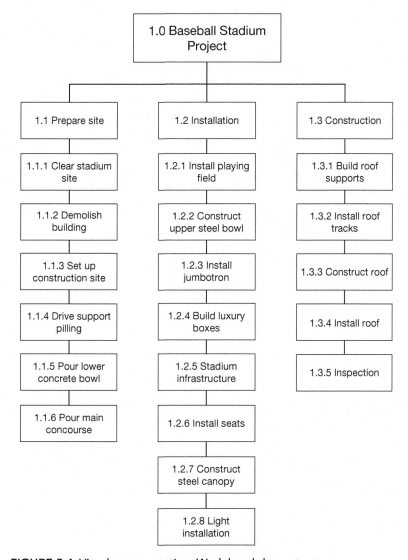

FIGURE 5.4 Visual representation: Work breakdown structure.

SOURCE: Sipes (2018).

It is important to know which tools should be developed first, then others may follow the same format, making each subsequent tool easier and more efficient to build. Project teams may struggle with the level of detail needed to use in the tools and documents; for example, the team might say it cannot develop the charter because it does not yet know enough about the project. It is important to remember that documents and tools developed are not set in stone and that changes can be made.

During this phase you may have the opportunity to see a demonstration of a new system. There should be a list of key questions about the potential new system for review; the vendors of the different systems must be open-minded and honest about the pros and cons of the system functionally.

CASE SCENARIO (CONTINUED)

Let's return to the case scenario. Camille is beginning to hear more about the new information system. Her manager is starting to share more information and is setting expectations of what all nurses can anticipate with the new system. One thing that really helped Camille and her colleagues get on board was the explanation of some of the new processes that will be used during the planning and implementation of the system.

When these were compared to the nursing process, which every nurse already knows, understands, and practices, their concerns began to be eased.

Especially important was the sharing of how the new system would benefit all nurses and make their jobs easier.

Camille has additional questions about her and her coworkers' roles in planning and designing the new system. She hears nurses will be needed to help test the new system.

1. Will there be any training on how to do this? What does it all mean?

2. How long will the testing take?

3. What will the nurses' role be if the system is not built according to the workflows they developed?

4. What is a super user? How will they be trained?

5. How will the patients be cared for during the times nurses have to help develop and implement the new system?

6. Discuss the nurses' role in the design and implementation of a new EHR. Why is it important for nurses to provide input into the design and workflow of the new system? Consider what would happen if IT developed the clinical documentation system without nurses' input into what is needed. What would be your response?

▦ Questions to Consider Before Reading on

1. *What is the value of using a project management process while working on a project or during clinical practice?*
2. *What is the nurse's role in testing the clinical system?*
3. *Why is it important for a nurse to understand and be involved in testing a new system?*
4. *Discuss different types of testing. What is the purpose of testing?*
5. *What does Acceptance Testing entail?*
6. *What is Usability Testing? What are the key components of Usability Testing and why is this testing important?*

Phase 3: Execution/Implementation

The third phase in project management is execution/implementation, which corresponds to the implementation phase of the nursing process. Project implementation or execution requires that everyone is involved, including the members of the nursing staff, and that all involved have explanations that enable them to understand the goal, expectations, and timeline. Nursing and project management go well together and many of their processes overlap.

As mentioned, during this third phase of project management, the project is executed/implemented (depending on the agency terminology). At this point, the tools previously developed will be used to start tracking project tasks and project activities that were outlined in the WBS. Whichever process best fits the project or activity, it is important to remember to use all of the planned steps.

As previously discussed, project management includes project initiation, planning, implementation, monitoring, and closing. Over time, project management has become useful in a variety of settings because it provides a structure and framework for completing tasks, and using systematic steps during project management can eliminate costly mistakes, increase quality, and save time, all with comparisons to the nursing process, as previously noted.

It is important to remember that a "project" is only a temporary activity, such as planning a wedding or developing a project for a graduate practicum, just as the steps in developing a patient care plan can be a temporary activity. One of the most important functions of a project is that of testing what was developed or created for clinicians' use. Unfortunately, when there is a time crunch in a project, testing is the one function that is cut back or eliminated.

Testing the System

The concept of testing is critically important. Remember the CNN News report which indicated (Payne, Smith, & Cohen, 2013) that "An internal government memo written just days before the start of open enrolment for Obamacare warned of a 'high' security risk because of a lack of testing of the HealthCare.gov website" (p. 1). CNN further reported, "officials of companies hired to create the HealthCare.gov website cited a lack of testing on the full system and last-minute changes by the federal agency overseeing the online enrolment system." Do you remember when the system first went "live"—it did not work and patients could not enroll in the system to get healthcare coverage?

Testing is typically broken down into a number of phases and designed to find errors and issues in the new system, called *bugs*, which must be corrected if the system is to work as designed. Testing should not be done just once; it is ongoing during the project management process, especially after the system is up and running. Systems are designed by application or module; each module or application is first tested individually. Depending on the testing process, the individual applications or modules are gradually integrated and then tested. Finally, all of the applications that have been tested and have passed are then moved into the entire system, where the system is then tested as a whole.

Nurses are involved in most testing, as well as in specific "acceptance or beta" testing, which is the final phase before implementation of a system and refers to whole-system testing during which final corrections are made, with the final step being implementation of the system the project designed. As a superuser or end user, you may be involved or have an opportunity to view the testing processes, which will provide valuable information and insight into how the process works, what works well, and what is not "user friendly" to your workflow.

You may also hear the term *usability testing*. The key principles of usability are simplicity, naturalness, consistency, minimizing cognitive load, efficient interactions, forgiveness and feedback, effective use of language, effective information presentation, and preservation of context (HIMSS, 2009). Testing for "usability" investigates how easy is it to use the keyboard and read the computer screen as well as how easy it is to click through the different tabs to find information. It is important to understand how this fits with testing, as many of these elements are incorporated into test scripts that you may use as a tester.

Testing is required to make sure everything that has been built works the way it was designed to work. There are many, many different types of testing; they cannot all be completed before a full system "goes live." Some of the more common terms associated with testing that you may be involved in are included in Box 5.3.

BOX 5.3

DIFFERENT TYPES OF TESTING OF NEW INFORMATION SYSTEMS

Unit testing. The "unit" being developed is tested during the building process.

Integration testing. These tests are completed to make sure the "unit" or application works with other units or applications—that it integrates well and does not cause problems.

System testing. This is a larger testing process used to verify that all of the applications across the system are tested. For example, do medication orders not only work well within the "order place" functionality, or do the orders flow to all of the areas where an order is needed?

Acceptance testing. This is a type of testing done by end users—those who will actually be using the application or system—to make sure it meets all expectations.

SOURCE: Shinde, V. (2012). What is the difference between unit testing and integration testing? Retrieved from https://www.softwaretestingclass.com/what-is-difference-between-unit-testing-and-integration -testing.

Again, there are many other types of testing, such as load testing, during which many users, especially nurses, are asked to complete a function, such as entering orders at the same time, to see whether the system slows down or even fails during a peak-use period. Another type of testing is usability testing, in which an end user works with the new system to determine how easy it is to use. There are many references on the web that can provide additional information on testing.

QSEN SCENARIO

You have been asked—as a superuser—to help test the new system to make sure everything is functioning correctly. What unique skills do you as a nurse bring to this that others will not have?

▨ Questions to Consider Before Reading on

1. *Discuss why monitoring and controlling a new system implementation are important.*

2. *What is the nurse's role in monitor and control as the new system is implemented?*

3. *Discuss why using metrics is important.*

4. *What is the nurse's role in closing the project and evaluating it after the new system is implemented?*

5. *Discuss why it is important to conduct a "lessons learned" assessment.*

Phase 4: Monitor/Control

Effective monitoring and control of a healthcare information system always involves tracking and gathering data about how something is functioning or what might need to be updated or even fixed. This is done through monitoring the metrics discussed earlier.

Metrics

There are different types of metrics. So what are metrics? Metrics can represent numbers of anything and are used as "standards of measurement by which efficiency, performance, progress, or quality of a plan, process, or product can be assessed" (BusinessDictionary .com, 2018; Sham, 2013).

Other types of metrics include more data known as *key performance indicators (KPIs)*, which you may have heard of. KPIs should also be tied to an objective; for example, this will be due on XXX or this rate will be reduced by XXX%, defined by specific objectives that answer the five Ws and an H (Sipes, 2016a), the who, what, where, when, why, and how.

Key to monitoring the project at this phase is to review the project plan on a regular basis, at least weekly, if not more frequently, to determine how the project is moving forward in terms of time, due dates, budget, scope, issues, and risks. Other objectives that will greatly impact the project require that the project be monitored from the very beginning of implementation to avoid surprises.

Phase 5: Closing/Evaluation

Closing a project can present a problem because it is sometimes difficult to find time to do this between the hectic schedule of finishing the previous project and having to move on to something else. If you were involved in the project, for example, helping to define workflows and then testing to make sure they are accurate with the new system, you must seamlessly transition the information you gained into the company's normal operations and "educate" the new person responsible for making sure everything works as designed. The final delivery of the "product" should be reviewed to make sure it meets the needs and expectations of the organization and end users.

During the closing phase, the tasks that need to be completed include debriefing the team, transitioning all of the appropriate documentation, and providing a project history as well as transitioning all activities back to those who will "own" and maintain them. The primary objective of the closing and transition processes is to obtain formal acceptance of the completed project by the project champion and key stakeholders, who are the end users (nurses), and other stakeholders who funded the project.

Lessons Learned

Lessons learned is a term frequently used after a project is completed. It is time to review, collect, and document information regarding how things went and what can be improved for the next project as well as to get feedback from everyone involved in the project. The lessons-learned session is usually set up in a meeting or conference room. Everyone involved is expected to attend and to contribute to the final assessment. All who have been involved in the project are invited to provide comment. One way this is done is to go around the table and have everyone share his or her insights while minutes are being recorded. After everyone has had a chance to provide input, data are collected and tabulated for the final report to be prepared. Things that need to be improved will be documented and assigned an owner in case there is a need for further resolution. The outcome of this meeting is to prepare a final report for leadership and stakeholders. Other objectives of the lessons learned function are provided in Box 5.4.

BOX 5.4

SUMMARY OF LESSONS LEARNED

- Define additional work that needs to be done.
- Determine whether there are other changes that need to be made to the project, and, if so, their processes or methodology.
- Define end user and key stakeholder satisfaction with the deliverable and the value and benefits of the project.
- Review the quality and performance of the project and teams.
- Ensure knowledge transfer with identified owners identified has occurred.

■ Critical Thinking Questions and Activities

- *You have been actively involved in the design and planning of the new EHR system that will be implemented in your healthcare facility. Other nurses were not as involved in the planning phase because they said they do not believe the new system is needed. How would you respond?*

- *Based on the previous question, what process would you employ to get other nurses more involved in developing the skills they need to be competent in using the new system?*

- *Consider the theory of Change Management described in Chapter 2. How would you apply these concepts to the scenario outlined in the first question? What process would you use?*

- *Work with your manager to prepare and present change management concepts to your co-workers.*

SUMMARY

This chapter introduced the concepts of project management and a subprocess, SDLC, as newer trends in nursing roles that are being developed; it discussed how project management relates to what you already know about the nursing process. The basics of project management were presented and an understanding given of how they correlate with the ANA's (2008) *Nursing Informatics: Scope and Standards of Practice*, and a discussion of how the processes can be useful as a framework for decision-making and critical thinking was presented.

The five phases of each process were presented and correlated to what you already know of the nursing process. Examples and diagrams were provided to add further explanation of the different processes many organizations use to track specific tasks. As the largest discipline providing patient care that uses EHRs, discussion of why nurses are needed to assist in the planning/design, implementation, testing, and evaluation of clinical systems was presented. Examples of the tasks that need to be completed during each phase and where nurses are needed in the process were presented.

■ References

American Library Association. (2014). Information literacy competency standards for nursing. Retrieved from crln.acrl.org/index.php/crlnews/article/download/9057/9901

American Nurses Association. (2008). *Nursing informatics: Scope and standards of practice.* Silver Spring, MD: Author.

American Nurses Association. (2015). *Nursing informatics: Scope and standards of practice* (3rd ed.). Silver Spring, MD: Author. Retrieved from https://www.nursingworld.org/practice-policy/scope-of-practice

American Recovery and Reinvestment Act. (2009). Medicaid and health care provisions. Retrieved from https://www.kff.org/medicaid/fact-sheet/american-recovery-and-reinvestment-act-arra-medicaid/

American Recovery and Reinvestment Act (ARRA, 2009). Recipient reporting. Frequently Asked Questions (FAQ). Retrieved from https://www.nsf.gov/bfa/dias/policy/arra/faqs_reportingmarch2014.pdf

American Recovery and Reinvestment Act (ARRA): Medicaid and Health Care Provisions. (2009). Capturing high quality electronic health records data. *HealthIT.gov.* Retrieved from www.healthit.gov/policy-researchers-implementers

BusinessDictionary.com. (2018). Metrics. Retrieved from http://www.businessdictionary.com/definition/metrics.html

Cunningham, C. (2018). Project life cycle (PLC) and system development life cycle (SDLC). Retrieved from neurontesting.blogspot.com/2012/06/project-life-cycle-plc-and-system.html

Health Information and Management Systems Society. (2009). Defining and testing EMR usability. Retrieved from www.himss.org/.../himssorg/.../HIMSSorg/.../HIMSS_DefiningandTestingEMRUsabilit

Health Information and Management Systems Society. (2014). Twenty-fifth Annual 2014 HIMSS leadership survey results. Retrieved from http://www.himss.org/25th-annual-2014-himss-leadership-survey-resultsh

Health IT Policy Committee: Recommendations to the National Coordinator. Retrieved from https://www.healthit.gov/.../health-it-policy-committee-recommendations-national-coordinator

HITECH Act Enforcement Interim Final. (2009). Retrieved from https://www.hhs.gov/hipaa/for-professionals/special-topics/hitech-act

Nightingale College. (2016). Goal setting for nursing learners: Learning the art of S.M.A.R.T. goals. Retrieved from https://nightingale.edu/blog/goal-setting-nursing-learners-learning-art-s-m-r-t-goals

Payne, E., Smith, M., & Cohen, T. (2013, October 22). Report: Healthcare website failed test ahead of rollout. *CNN.* Retrieved from https://www.cnn.com/2013/10/22/politics/obamacare-website-problems/index.html

Project Management Institute. (2017). A guide to the project management body of knowledge (PMBOK® guide, 6th ed.). Newtown Square, PA: Author.

Project Management Institute. (2018). What is project management? Retrieved from https://www.pmi.org/about/learn-about-pmi/what-is-project-management

Sham, K. (2013). *Practical approach to project management metrics.* Paper presented at PMI® Global Congress 2013—North America, New Orleans, LA. Newtown Square, PA: Project Management Institute.

Shinde, V. (2012). What is the difference between unit testing and integration testing? Retrieved from https://www.softwaretestingclass.com/what-is-difference-between-unit-testing-and-integration-testing

Sipes, C. (2016a). *Project management for the advance practice nurse.* New York, NY: Springer Publishing.

Sipes, C. (2016b). Project management: Essential skill of nurse informaticists. *Studies in Health Technology and Informatics, 225,* 252–256. doi:10.3233/978-1-61499-658-3-252

Sipes, C., Hunter, K., McGonigle, D., Hebda, T., Hill, T., & Lamblin J. (2016).Competency skills assessment: Successes and areas for improvement identified during collaboration between informaticists and a national organization. *Studies in Health Technology and Informatics, 225,* 43–47. doi:10.3233/978-1-61499-658-3-43

CHAPTER 6

NURSING INFORMATICS: RESEARCH APPLICATIONS

CAROLYN SIPES

LEARNING OBJECTIVES AND OUTCOMES

Upon completion of this chapter, the reader will be able to:

- Define *nursing research*.
- Discuss the bachelor of science in nursing (BSN) role in nursing research utilization.
- Define differences between qualitative and quantitative research.
- Discuss how you use computer literacy to develop a research agenda.
- Discuss why nursing informatics is important. List one research or practice outcome in which nursing informatics skills are applied.
- List four nursing informatics competencies identified in the ANA position statement expected of the baccalaureate nurse.

⊙ KEY NURSING INFORMATICS TERMS

Key concepts and terms you will hear in the discipline of nursing informatics are:

Agency for Healthcare Research and Quality (AHRQ)

Canadian/American Spinal Research Organizations (CSRO/ASRO)

Competencies

Computer literacy

Correlation

Data collection

Data management

Database search

eHealth

Evidence-based practice (EBP)

MEDLINE

⊙ **KEY NURSING INFORMATICS TERMS** (*continued*)

National Institute for Nursing Research (NINR)

Nursing informatics research

Nursing research

Patient-centered outcomes research (PCOR)

Peer reviewed

Qualitative research

Quantitative research

Seminal works

Technological evolution

World Wide Web (www)

INTRODUCTION: RESEARCH ESSENTIALS

What are some of your experiences using research at work in your clinical practice and in your nursing program? Have you been involved in a research project or assisted with data collection during which you used computer technology to gather patient information?

Consider some of the general experiences you have in your current practice environment. How have you used research in your job role? Did you have to look up information related to the patient care you provided to find a best practice? Was the information relevant and current and evidence based? How long did it take you to find the information using the computer versus going to the library to complete a search?

The experiences related to what you may already know from your practice and have learned from the nursing program will provide answers to these questions. These questions may also stimulate curiosity about how you can further develop research skills and understanding that can provide answers to many practice questions or identify more questions you might like to explore with your own research project and the evidence you need to be able to provide EBP.

▦ Questions to Consider Before Reading On

1. *What are the differences between qualitative and quantitative research?*
2. *What was the study method in the qualitative research study Exemplar 1?*
3. *What conclusion was drawn from the qualitative research study Exemplar 1?*
4. *What was the background/reason for conducting the qualitative research study Exemplar 2?*

▦ What Is Nursing Research?

The basic definition of *research* means "to search again" or "investigate" in order to understand and gain new knowledge or refine existing knowledge, or in the case of nursing, to improve patient care and clinical practice. Research in nursing means to search for evidence unique to and supportive of the discipline of nursing and its practice. As nurses work with patients every day, they have opportunities to see problems that could be solved through investigation and to make recommendations for changes based on research investigating how to find a better way to practice and improve care. To research is to ask questions based on personal experiences and knowledge that can be explored and to integrate findings into practice in order to improve patient care, regardless of practice area. The National Institute of Nursing Research (NINR, 2016) defines nursing research as foundational to developing knowledge to:

- Build the scientific foundation for clinical practice.
- Prevent disease and disability.
- Manage and eliminate symptoms caused by illness.
- Enhance end-of-life and palliative care.

There are some important definitions used to explain the components and characteristics of nursing research, but first we need the definition of *nursing*. The American Nurses Association (ANA) definition of *nursing* is as follows:

> *Nursing is the protection, promotion, and optimization of health and abilities, prevention of illness and injury, facilitation of healing, alleviation of suffering through the diagnosis and treatment of human response, and advocacy in the care of individuals, families, groups, communities, and populations.* (ANA, 2018, p. 1)

Nursing informatics (NI) research is another concept that continues to grow. Originally described by Effken (2003) as a model connecting nursing and informatics in order to study the practice of NI, today, that practice includes the use of technology to pull vast amounts of information from electronic health records (EHRs) and other sources.

As a foundation of nursing knowledge discussed in other chapters in this book, and in terms of understanding and applying the data–information-knowledge–wisdom (DIKW) process, research is based on a good idea, theory, or understanding of the research process, and use of tools and resources. It involves deciding whether the good lead is a researchable question and then refining the idea into a research question. It also includes determining ways to capture the data relevant to the question, analyzing the results, and then disseminating the findings to the larger nursing population.

Most of the searches for evidence today are done with the use of computers. More about the use of computers and development of computer literacy will be provided in the following chapters.

Questions to Consider Before Reading On

1. *Reflecting on your own level of competency, what do you already know and what have you learned from the previous chapters that is new information?*
2. *Going forward, reflecting on a self-assessment, what do you need to know?*

Categories of Nursing Research—Qualitative

Before starting an investigation or research we need to understand the different categories of research and how each applies to a specific problem identified to be studied.

The most familiar categories of research you may have experience with are qualitative research and quantitative research, defined in the next section. Within each category are different types of research.

The goal of this text is not to develop researchers, but to provide an overview of the different research processes and an explanation of how NI and computer use and literacy are foundational and integral to research.

Qualitative Research

Qualitative research is defined as an approach used to generate knowledge that employs methods of inquiry that emphasize subjectivity by describing and giving meaning to the experience. According to Denzin and Lincoln (2011), a key feature of qualitative research is to find meaning in the same way that study participations assign it to a particular phenomenon under study. According to the CSRO/ASRO, qualitative research uses an unstructured form of data collection that tries to find answers to questions regarding human behavior and is characterized by questions that ask why or how (CSRO/ASRO, 2015).

For example, when selecting a topic, one participant might assign a different meaning to being "overweight" or "overeating" than another. To investigate this phenomenon further, the type of framework or study design needs to be identified based on the question or problem. Next, the importance of the study must be justified; identification of data sources such as who will be in the study group, determination of how and what data to collect are completed.

The final steps in the process require intensive use of technology and NI skills for data to be collected and managed, which requires description, analysis, and interpretation of the information to be able to assign meaning to the research topic, then publish the final report.

Types of qualitative research include: defining data-collection methods used: observation, interviews, ethnographic study, grounded theory, phenomenology, and examining written text. Consider which type of qualitative research you might use in the prior example. Should it be observation, interviews, ethnography, grounded theory, phenomenology, or examining written text?

CASE SCENARIOS—QUALITATIVE RESEARCH EXEMPLARS

EXEMPLAR 1

Study Statement: The qualitative study participants involved 60 nurses from five countries (Canada, India, Ireland, Japan, and Korea) who took part in 11 focus groups that discussed the question: Do you consider your work meaningful? Fostering meaning and mentorship as part of the institutional culture was a central theme that emerged from the discussions.
Methods: Researchers first defined the meaning of *meaningful work* as presented in the literature related to existentialism and hardiness. Second, they defined the method and analysis used in the study, asking how nurses find meaning in their very challenging work, and then reported findings of four themes that emerged from the comments shared by nurses,

(continued)

(continued)

specifically, relationships, compassionate caring, identity, and a mentoring culture. Findings and the limitations of the qualitative study were documented.

Conclusion: The conclusion was that nursing leaders and a culture of mentorship play an important role in fostering meaningful work and developing hardy employees (Malloy et al. 2015).

EXEMPLAR 2

Study Statement: Nurses strive to provide holistic care, including spiritual care, for all patients. However, in busy critical care environments, nurses often feel driven to focus on patients' physical care, possibly at the expense of emotional and spiritual care. This study examined how Palestinian nurses working in intensive care units (ICUs) understand spirituality and the provision of spiritual care at the end of life.

Background: This study encouraged an increased emphasis on spiritual care.

Method: Qualitative research was used to study 13 ICU Gaza Strip nurses' understanding of spiritual care.

Findings: The following themes were identified: meaning of spirituality and spiritual care, identifying spiritual needs, and taking actions to meet spiritual needs.

Discussion/Limitations: Nurses had difficulty in differentiating spiritual and religious needs.

Conclusion: Recommendations were made for increased emphasis on the provision of spiritual care for all patients (Abu-El-Noor, 2016).

Critical Thinking Questions and Activities

1. *As you read through the studies, what questions would you still want to explore yet if the studies were to continue?*

2. *What would you take from this to apply to your practice?*

3. *What would you do differently if this were your study?*

Questions to Consider Before Reading On

1. *What study method was used in the quantitative research study?*

2. *What type of technology was evaluated?*

3. *What conclusion was drawn from the quantitative research study? Would you be able to replicate this type of study in your practice?*

Categories of Nursing Research—Quantitative

Quantitative Research

Quantitative research is defined as a formal, objective, rigorous approach to the generation of knowledge based on determining how a given behavior, characteristics, or phenomenon is present. This type of research examines cause and effect and requires the ability to replicate the study in order to demonstrate reliability, validity, and rigor, which is sometimes called *systematic inquiry*. Again, computers and other technology are used extensively to conduct these research studies.

Quantitative research is used extensively in both natural and social sciences. Unlike qualitative research, this type of research is concerned with numerical measurements and statistics (Yarcheski & Mahon, 2013). Often, standardized instruments are used as part of a structured methodology of data collection. Quantitative research focuses on asking questions that pertain to what, where, or when? There are six main types of study designs in quantitative research.

When defining a quantitative research problem, the significance of the issue must first be determined. For example, are patients' falls an issue at your organization? To develop a research study to explore this problem, you would need to consider the following questions.

- What are the potential outcomes and consequences if the number of falls increases over a given period of time?
- Using technology, how and where would you search for data and other information?
- Would you search databases from national organizations such as the AHRQ?
- What different types of analysis would you need to conduct?
- Would you use a software program to code data?
- Would data need to be displayed in a certain way such as with bar charts and graphs?
- What type of statistical analysis would be required using computational software?
- How and where would you store your data and other research information using technology?

Types of quantitative research include: descriptive, correlational, quasi-experimental, and experimental. The type of research is determined by the research problem that is developed and existing reach of that problem.

CASE SCENARIO—QUANTITATIVE STUDY

EXEMPLAR 1

Healthcare workers in this qualitative research example used smartphones, something every nurse today can identify with. Remember that quantitative research focuses on asking questions that pertain to what, where, or when? This cross-sectional survey example meets the criteria that the researchers observe what is happening without interfering. Data are collected at a specific point in time and often used to assess the prevalence of an illness or disease.

Study Statement: Mobile phone applications are useful for addressing challenges and improving the quality of data collection in developing countries.

(continued)

(continued)

> *Method:* A cross-sectional observational study using a structured paper checklist was prepared to assess the completeness and accuracy of electronic records over a period of 6 months. When compared to paper records, the use of electronic forms significantly improved data completeness. *Results:* Of entries checked for completeness, 99.2% of electronic record entries were complete. *Conclusion:* With minimal training, supervision, and no incentives, healthcare workers were able to use electronic forms for patient assessment and routine data collection appropriately and accurately with a very small error rate (Medhanyie et al., 2017).

Critical Thinking Questions and Activities – Quantitative Exemplar

1. *As you read through this quantitative study, would you be able to conduct the study in the same way using smartphones?*
2. *While this research study was conducted in a developing country, what similarities do you see that might apply to your practice environment in the US?*
3. *What other types of technology could you use to collect data?*

Questions to Consider Before Reading On

1. *Why is research important to nursing?*
2. *List two scenarios in which you could apply nursing research in your current practice from the healthcare areas listed in the next section.*
3. *Where would we be if there was no way to conduct research to search for the best practice models using technology?*
4. *How and what would you do to find out how other nurses practice using research to support practice?*

Why Is Research Important to Nurses?

The first time nurses might be introduced to the concept of nursing research is in a BSN degree program. There they will explore concepts, different types of nursing research, and how these then apply to a particular investigation searching for an answer to a question or problem, which can then be applied to practice. Blake (2016), in the article, "Yes, Nurses Do Research, and It's Improving Patient Care," suggests that nurses need to get involved in research to build a solid base of evidence, to search for answers to healthcare problems so as to provide more effective practices using NI skills and tools to search and retrieve important data and information for research studies. The goal should not only be those of helping patients and families, but also collaborating with interprofessional teams in hospitals.

Research is needed to develop scientific knowledge. As discussed, different categories and types of research are needed in order to develop best practices based on inquiry and application of evidence. Research can provide important information about many aspects of healthcare. For example, exploring other practices through research can provide information regarding many areas of healthcare, including:

- Disease trends
- Risk factors
- Outcomes of treatment
- Public health interventions
- Functional abilities
- Patterns of care
- Healthcare costs and use

Today, healthcare is constantly changing, especially with our technology-rich practice environments. This means with changes, clinical practice needs to constantly be evaluated to further improve the quality of care provided. Scientific knowledge can be developed through use of nursing research to improve healthcare and outcomes for patients, which is the main goal of nursing investigation and EBP (Despins & Wakefield, 2018). But once the scientific knowledge is developed, how is it applied to practice? (For an example of the process, see Figure 6.1.)

QSEN SCENARIO

Sue has learned a number of ways that research is important to nursing by following and observing a peer more experienced in research. She identified a problem while taking care of a patient in the ICU and would like to find out more about this patient's diagnosis and possible newer treatment modalities, but is not sure what questions to ask or even where to look if she were to use the computer for an electronic literature search.

1. Do you know how to ask the right questions?
2. Do you know how to conduct an electronic literature search to find the answers?
3. What are some potential benefits of using nursing research in your practice?

■ Questions to Consider Before Reading On

1.   *What are some ways NI and nursing research are linked?*
2.   *How can you best continue to develop your knowledge base using NI and other technology to support research?*
3.   *What are some activities you will be involved in to accomplish this?*
4.   *What are four roles a BSN and all nurses with NI knowledge and skills can assume?*
5.   *How did mandates and research agendas from national organizations impact the universal requirement to advance use of healthcare technology, knowledge, and skills in nursing?*
6.   *What are three of the major nursing organizations?*

Linking Nursing Informatics and Research

In Chapter 1, you learned that *NI* is defined as nursing science that integrates "data information, knowledge, and wisdom in nursing practice" (ANA, 2015, p. 2) and that the use of technology is extensive and every aspect of nursing practice falls within the category of informatics nurse (ANA, 2015). Can you think of an example of how this might apply to you?

The ANA includes the advancement of outcomes for population health in their informatics framework (ANA, 2015). When nurses have a degree of informatics proficiency, they are better equipped to manage patients' complex medical data and to problem solve through research in order to provide high-quality patient care, to support consumers and the interprofessional healthcare team in their decision-making in all roles and settings to achieve desired outcomes.

Nursing informaticists work as developers of information structures, information processes, and information technology (IT) to advance healthcare. As discussed earlier, NI is very relevant to nursing research through the use of technology as it has evolved into an expanding body of knowledge, confirming and supporting its relevance and applicability to all domains of nursing, including research, practice, information management, and technology (Hunter & Bickford, 2015).

As discussed in Chapter 2, the Quality and Safety Education for Nurses (QSEN) initiative defined six key areas of knowledge, skills, and attitudes (KSAs) competencies in nursing prelicensure and BSN programs, including those for NI education (Cronenwett et al., 2009). As seen in Box 6.1, a number of the KSAs link NI, the use of technology, information, and research activities as discussed previously, such as searching databases and using information management tools.

BOX 6.1

QUALITY AND SAFETY EDUCATION FOR NURSES

KNOWLEDGE, SKILLS, AND ATTITUDES—PREPARING FUTURE NURSES

Informatics defined: Use of information and technology to communicate, manage knowledge, mitigate error, and support decision-making (QSEN, 2018)

Explain why information and technology skills are essential for safe patient care (knowledge)

Identify essential information that must be available in a common database to support patient care (knowledge)

Navigate the electronic health record; document and plan patient care in an electronic health record (skills)

Value technologies that support clinical decision-making, error prevention, and care coordination (attitudes)

(continued)

BOX 6.1 (continued)

KNOWLEDGE, SKILLS, AND ATTITUDES—PREPARING FUTURE NURSES

Describe examples of how technology and information management are related to the quality and safety of patient care; recognize the time, effort, and skill required for computers, databases, and other technologies to become reliable and effective tools for patient care (knowledge)

Respond appropriately to clinical decision-making supports and alerts, use information management tools to monitor outcomes of care processes, and use high-quality electronic sources of healthcare information (skills)

Value nurses' involvement in design, selection, implementation, and evaluation of information technologies to support patient care (attitudes)

SOURCE: Adapted from Cronenwett, L., Sherwood, G., Barnsteiner, J., Disch, J., Johnson, J., Mitchell P., ... Warren, J. (2007). Quality and Safety Education for Nurses. *Nursing Outlook, 55*(3), 122–131. doi:10.1016/j. outlook.2007.02.006.

The context for NI research has changed significantly since the NINR funded the NI research agenda. This organization mandated that an NI research agenda for 2008 through 2018 must expand all users of interest in activities related to NI and research. What follows is a partial list of mandates (NINR, 2016):

- Build on the knowledge gained in nursing concept definitions to address genomic and environmental data; for example, transforming and applying new treatment options such as cancer treatments.

- Guide the reengineering of nursing practice; for example, all nurses increased their application and knowledge of technology in all practice areas.

- Harness new technologies to empower patients and their caregivers to collaborate on knowledge development; for example, nurses assist patients in accessing their health records through patient portals.

- Develop user-configurable software approaches that support complex data visualization, analysis, and predictive modeling; for example, expand use of smartphones and other devices.

- Encourage innovative evaluation methodologies using a human–computer interface and an organizational context; for example, nurses demonstrated advanced use of mouse, keyboards, touch screens, and other devices that plug into the computer.

In 2016, the NINR further developed a strategic plan identifying specific future directions for nurses to follow to link more use of technology called *Technology to Improve Health*. It recognized that "accelerating availability and accessibility of innovative technologies provide nursing science with an ideal opportunity to reach diverse and underserved populations, improving health and preventing illness across the lifespan" (p. 23).

Using multiple technology systems to support research, the NINR will prioritize research to:

- Identify the essential components of successful, evidence-based, innovative interventions that are easily tailored to diverse population groups across healthcare settings.

- Support interprofessional research and nursing informaticists to develop system infrastructures by building partnerships with technical developers (e.g., engineers and designers) and communities to design and test new technologies in various settings.

- Develop technologies to maximize the use of innovative methodologies to integrate the community's voice and cultural perspectives to promote positive health behaviors and manage chronic conditions across conditions, communities, and ages.

- Explore a wide range of technological formats (e.g., video/audio, data-collection tools, smart devices, telehealth) that can be used to improve the cultural similarities of health interventions to improve health for all. (NINR, 2016)

BOX 6.2

LINKING NURSING INFORMATICS TO THE RESEARCH PROCESS TO EXPAND EVIDENCE

One example: The *what is* and *how to* of understanding application of the research process and its importance to nursing includes steps such as:

1. While providing patient care on the medical–surgical unit, a problem in patient care is identified, but there are no current processes in place to address the issue.

2. Using technology and searching databases for the latest EBPs and outcomes are initiated to find support for the current best practice. This is done based on practice experience, collecting and documenting evidence using technology, asking questions—the how, what, and why—then formulating a hypothesis and offering considerations for possible applications and outcomes based on evidence.

3. Based on the evidence, a process is developed to address the specific patient problem.

4. Finally, evaluation of the outcomes is completed, leading to new developments, improvements, and education so as to provide best practices through application of the EBP.

5. A final step is to develop a procedure to use to address the problem going forward.

Questions to Consider Before Reading On

1. *When considering a clinical problem, what is the first step in assessing the problem?*

2. *After you have determined what the problem is, how will you find the answers to your clinical question?*

As discussed in Chapter 1, the ANA's *Nursing Informatics: Scope and Standards of Practice* lists specific standards that link NI to nursing research; these are Standard 9, Evidence-Based Practice, and Standard 10: Research Quality of Practice (ANA, 2015). There are many other competencies outside of Standard 9 that are incorporated into clinical practice that also apply to nursing research and these are the expected, basic informatics levels and skills for all nurses, including prelicensure and BSN nurses. Again, the complete list of standards can be found in Chapter 1.

The American Association of Colleges of Nursing (AACN) Essentials, also discussed in Chapter 1, also identified essentials that specifically link NI and nursing research. Included are:

- Essential III—Scholarship for Evidence Based Practice
- Essential IV—Information Management and Application of Patient Care Technology
- Essential IX—Baccalaureate Generalist Nursing Practice

Competency examples are also provided with the definitions of the standards.

Questions to Consider Before Reading On

1. *Discuss a research challenge you might expect in the future.*
2. *How will informatics and technology link EBP and research?*
3. *How is patient-centered outcomes research (PCOR) different from what and how practice is today?*

Newer Research Challenges for the 2025 Workforce

Risling (2017) suggests that the pace of technological evolution in healthcare is rapidly advancing. Student nurses, and those already in practice, should be offered ongoing educational opportunities to enhance a wide spectrum of professional informatics skills, including learning and applying the concepts of linking EBP and research through the application of informatics and technology with the use of electronic literature searches. A key consideration is that nurses of the 2025 workforce will most certainly inhabit a very different practice environment than what exists today, and technology will be key to this transformation (Risling, 2017).

Today, there is a new term used in healthcare: *e-Health (electronic health) care,* which was necessitated by the increased use of technology in electronic health and medical records included for all nursing patients in all phases of healthcare. The goal of these new concepts is to get patients more involved in their healthcare decisions; it generated a new type of research: PCOR. This dramatic change in healthcare research emerged with a focus on patient-centered outcomes research (PCOR).

According to the AHRQ (2013), when reviewing recent evidence on standard medical metrics (mortality and morbidity), "it was noted that metrics and outcomes of particular interest to patients and families (such as quality of life) were understudied (pp. 1–2)" and a need was identified requiring evidence on patient-centered outcomes from the perspective of the patient. A new institute was formed with the following mission:

> *The Patient-Centered Outcomes Research Institute (PCORI) helps people make informed health care decisions, and improves health care delivery and outcomes, by producing and promoting high integrity, evidence-based information that comes from research guided by patients, caregivers and the broader health care community.* (PCORI, 2013, para. 1)

These calls to action encourage early and meaningful engagement of patients and other stakeholders, such as nurses, at all levels of practice, in stating the research question, conducting the study, and interpreting the results (AHRQ, 2013). This new direction in healthcare research will produce evidence that is coinvestigated by patients and families in partnership with nurses, increasing its relevance so that EBPs reflect the patients' viewpoint. According to Newhouse, Barksdale, and Miller (2015), goals of nursing research are well aligned with PCORI interests and provide ongoing research opportunities to improve patient-centered outcomes of care.

Questions to Consider Before Reading On

1. *What are two basic skills needed in clinical practice to provide and use evidence in practice and support of patients by using NI skills and technology?*
2. *What are important steps to take to find and evaluate the best evidence for practice?*
3. *What are four recommendations of basic competencies needed by all nurses?*

Linking Evidence-Based Practice and Research

Many of the skills and knowledge needed to acquire and integrate research findings into practice have been discussed previously. Expectations of the 2025 workforce and definitions and examples of different categories and types of research have been presented.

There are many different definitions of *evidence based practice*. Evidence based practice (EBP) is defined as a problem-solving approach to clinical decision-making within a healthcare organization. It integrates the best available scientific evidence with the best available experiential (patient and practitioner) evidence (Oregon Health & Science University Library, 2018). It is based on principles that, with practitioner expertise and support, better research findings lead to patients' better clinical decision-making where their values and preferences are considered key in the decision-making process. This requires that the practitioner be information literate in that the healthcare provider—usually the nurse—understands how, where, and what the most current and valid research findings are. The process for appraising and finding the best evidence is presented in Figure 6.1.

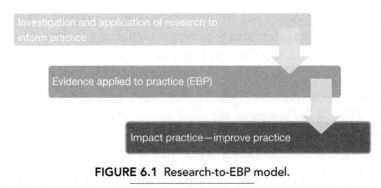

FIGURE 6.1 Research-to-EBP model.

EBP, evidence-based practice.

SOURCE: Sipes (2018).

The ability to locate relevant information to guide clinical practice is important for both quality nursing care and patient safety. *The Future of Nursing: Leading Change, Advancing Health* (Institute of Medicine, 2015) supports and recommends that skills and education are needed by *all* nurses in the new high-tech healthcare environment. Today, patient healthcare needs and care have become more complex, but many times nurses' knowledge, skills, and competencies have not kept up with the changes required to provide a safer, high-quality, high-tech healthcare.

Included in the recommendations of basic competencies needed by all nurses is the ability to use technology by using NI skills to:

■ Collect evidence-based research (EBR) to apply to improve practice

■ Develop information and computer literacy skills in order to effectively use an EHR, technology, and other clinical systems

■ Create healthcare polices through data collection

■ Develop specific competencies related to the areas of practice such as

  ○ Telehealth in community health

  ○ Use of medical devices in all clinical practice areas

With high-tech practice and use of EHRs, nurses with computer skills and an understanding of informatics are needed to facilitate communication with other interdisciplinary teams as well as IT.

In addition, the IOM report noted other areas in which informatics competencies are needed, these include workforce planning and policy making based on research and data collection, all of which require technology, computers, and information literacy.

Further supported by ANA Standard 9 discussed earlier, the "informatics nurse integrates evidence and research findings into practice" (ANA, 2015, p. 83), citing tasks to link EBP and research competencies, including:

■ Discussing how the evidence should be identified and collected

■ Integrating evidence into practice will initiate change

■ Improving care processes and decisions

- Guiding practice
- Disseminating findings to peers
- Applying informatics skills and tools in order to participate and conduct research studies appropriate for BSN-level education.

The process of EBP involves a systematic process into many areas of research to find the relevant answer to a practice question and support clinical decision making. (Stevens, 2013)

Questions to Consider Before Reading On

1. *What is computer literacy?*
2. *How can nurses be effectively supported to use evidence from research?*
3. *What are questions to explore in order to find relevant and current research to apply in clinical practice?*

Computer Literacy, Information, and Research Used to Develop Evidence-Based Practice

Selected *Essentials of Baccalaureate Education* were presented in Chapter 1, which emphasized that the translation of evidence into practice for professional nursing practice, known as *EBP*, is sorely needed (AACN, 2008). Foundational competencies, such as computer and information literacy, are key to improving quality and safety of nursing practice. As discussed earlier, computers are used for many functions, including searching for information and research to discover and support EBP.

Computer literacy—the proficient use of computers and other technological equipment—is a core competency needed in healthcare and nursing practice and should be taught in nursing curricula at all levels. In addition, information literacy—the ability to identify and find, evaluate, organize, and use information effectively—must be integrated into practice and used to support knowledge management (ANA, 2015). According to the ANA (2015), the following competencies are essential for *all* beginning nurses:

- Basic computer literacy, including the ability to use basic desktop applications and electronic communication
- The ability to use IT to support clinical and administrative processes, which presumes information literacy to support EBP
- The ability to access data and perform documentation via computerized patient records
- The ability to support patient safety initiatives via the use of IT

Information literacy forms the basis of lifelong learning. It is common to all disciplines, to all learning environments, and to all levels of education. It enables learners to master content and extend their investigations, become more self-directed, and assume greater control over their own learning. Information literacy is the set of skills needed to understand, find, retrieve, analyze, and use information (Association of College & Research Libraries, 2014).

Issue: Lack of Skills Needed to Conduct Research-Based Evidence-Based Practice

Melnyk, Fineout-Overholt, Gallagher-Ford, and Kaplan (2012) found nurses valued and implemented EBP and sought structured education and guidance to improve their use of evidence in practice. However, many faced barriers, including lack of time, lack of EBP knowledge, need for more education, no access to evidence, and resistance from colleagues or managers. Melnyk, Gallagher-Ford, Long, and Fineout-Overholt (2014) provided strategies for the integration of EBP into nursing organizations that focus on promoting a culture of EBP, establishing performance expectations, and sustaining EBP activities. As discussed in their previous study, Melnyk et al. (2012) identified that a key component for EBP was scheduling time for nurse engagement.

Based on Melnyk et al.'s (2012, 2014) research and in order for nurses to effectively use evidence, they must be supported and:

- Provided the environment, time, and resources to ask clinical questions and engage with mentors in a literature review, evidence synthesis, and data collection or interpretation

- Provided the mentorship and support to obtain continuing education about how to engage in EBP and about implementing EBP change

- Aware of available resources to learn more about EBP and about how to carry out EBP at the institutional level

These are recommendations presented in studies; the overall consensus is that future research is needed to evaluate the best approach to improving EBP.

Skills needed to be successful were further emphasized by Melnyk et al.'s study 2014. As more emphasis is placed on the ability to find research to support EBP using today's technology, other reports have found that advances in technology have changed how students access evidence-based information. Long et al. (2016) found that students overestimate their ability to locate quality online research and lack the skills needed to evaluate scientific literature. Clinical nurses report relying on personal experience to answer clinical questions rather than searching evidence-based sources. To address the problem, a web-based EBR tool that is usable from a computer, smartphone, or tablet was developed and tested. The purpose of the EBR tool is to guide students through the basic steps needed to locate and critically appraise the online scientific literature while linking users to quality electronic resources to support EBP (Long et al., 2016).

Response to Issues

As noted, there is movement to address these issues as in the Long et al. (2016) study, in which they developed a tool to help guide students to locate scientific literature (see reference list to access this study). In response to need, educators are developing courses that incorporate and offer opportunities to develop skills in simulation, virtual worlds, and provide exercises in searching for evidence.

Finding the Literature

Finding the most current, relevant, and reliable research literature can be a challenge. There are library resources and electronic literature searches that require a computer and current Internet access; the most commonly used browser is the World Wide Web. Peer-reviewed scholarly literature for healthcare can be found on databases and indexes, such as MEDLINE, Cumulative Index of Nursing and Allied Health Literatiure (CINAHL), the Cochran Library, as well as others, including those that offer patient teaching materials such as MedlinePlus.

The skills needed and questions to ask when searching the literature include:

- Which database will you search? Remember there are many resources, and searches should not be limited to just the library or the Internet.

- Is the literature current and relevant? What is the publication date? It should be within the past 5 years unless it is a seminal work. Define the publication date limit where you expect to find the most current and relevant information. Seminal works are frequently cited by other and older, original, foundational works.

- What is the quality and quantity of the information returned? Relevant searches should return no more than 50 items.

- Is the information peer reviewed or otherwise evaluated?

- What is your skill in sorting and using keywords or subject headings of articles?

QSEN SCENARIO

You may have to search several systems to complete a bibliographic retrieval. Many of the sites have directions for ways to use the World Wide Web, for example, www .ncbi.nlm.nih.gov/pubmed/ is used for a PubMed search; and www.ncbi.nlm.nih.gov/ mesh is used for MeSH (medical subject headings), the U.S. National Library of Medicine's controlled vocabulary for indexing articles for MEDLINE/PubMed. These are examples of bibliographic retrieval systems.

1. Why would you search any of these sites? What would you expect to find?

CASE SCENARIO

Kathy has been working in the ICU, caring for a patient diagnosed with atrial fibrillation and she is in the process of ruling out a cerebral vascular accident (CVA). Kathy has many questions about how to find the most current EBP and standards in caring for a patient with this diagnosis. She has had some experience using NI skills to define and use database searches, but has not done so in a long time. She asks her manager what she should do. Her manager directs her to the PubMed site, Quick Start (www.ncbi.nlm.nih.gov/books/NBK3827/#pubmedhelp .PubMed_Quick_Start) and suggests Kathy start by reviewing the YouTube tutorial so that she will know how to complete an electronic literature search.

(continued)

(continued)

Kathy begins to conduct her search for the information, but is not sure where to start. Questions she considers:

1.   First things first, what exactly am I looking for? To create a list?
2.   What are the topics I should use so I can narrow my search?

After completing the Quick Start tutorial, Kathy finds there are many other areas she can explore within the same link if she clicks on more tabs at the www.ncbi.nlm.nih.gov site, including www.ncbi.nlm.nih.gov/pubmedhealth/s/full_text_reviews medrev/, where she will find the full-text articles she is looking for.

3.   Next she asks how to retrieve the documents and information she needs.
4.   How can she download the information or print it?

■ Question to Consider Before Reading On

   1.   If you had no literature-search experience, where would you begin to gain experience in searches?

E-Literature Searches

Selected examples and tools of some of the more frequently used retrieval systems as well as how to complete a database search are included in this section. The best place to start to develop electronic literature skills and to begin a search is with a YouTube tutorial, as you can see in Figure 6.2.

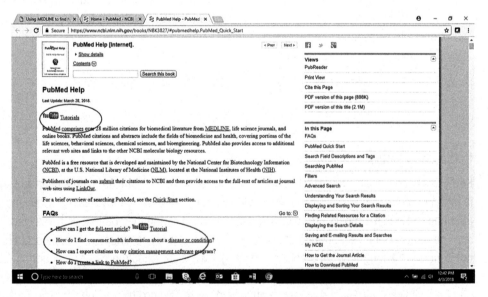

FIGURE 6.2

SOURCE: U.S. National Library of Medicine. (2018f). PubMed quick start. Retrieved from https://www.ncbi.nlm.nih .gov/books/NBK3827/#pubmedhelp.PubMed_Quick_Start.

As you use the Quick Start tutorial, you will learn how to search for the information you need; then as you become more comfortable and explore more, you can attempt to get the *full-text articles,* for example, or search for a *specific disease* (U.S. National Library of Medicine, 2018f).

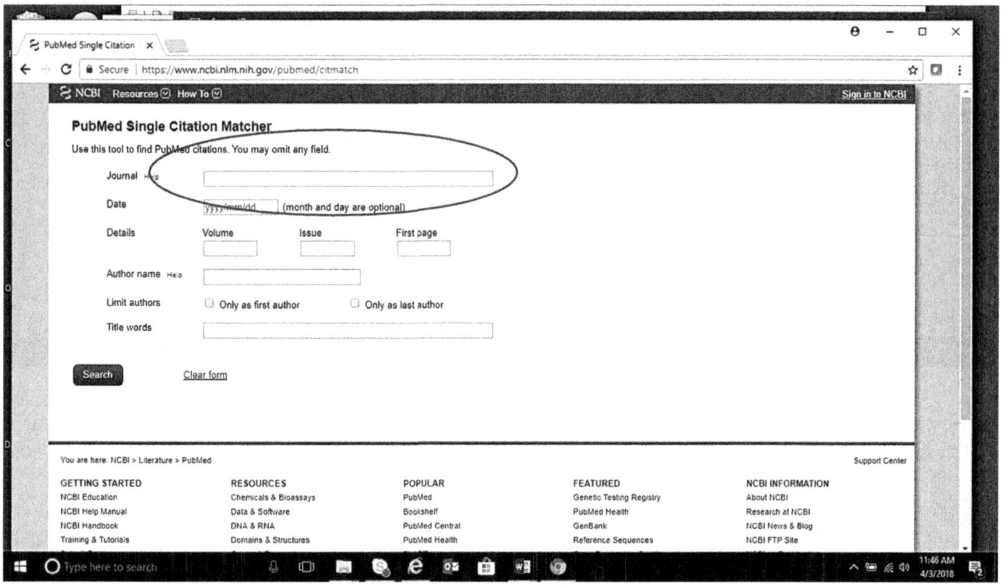

FIGURE 6.3

SOURCE: U.S. National Library of Medicine. (2018e). PubMed. Retrieved from https://www.ncbi.nlm.nih.gov/pubmed.

After you have completed the tutorials mentioned, move on to other ways of finding the information you need. In Figure 6.3, there is a field to complete if you are searching for a specific journal, authors, or a title you may want to find.

MeSH is the U.S. National Library of Medicine's controlled vocabulary for indexing articles for MEDLINE/PubMed (Figure 6.4). MeSH terminology provides a consistent way to retrieve information that may use different terms for the same concepts.

One of the benefits of using MeSH terms is that when you search with them, you get all the articles about a topic, regardless of what term the authors used. If you are unsure of how to navigate the site, be sure to take advantage of the tutorials; also note the other resources highlighted on the left of Figure 6.4.

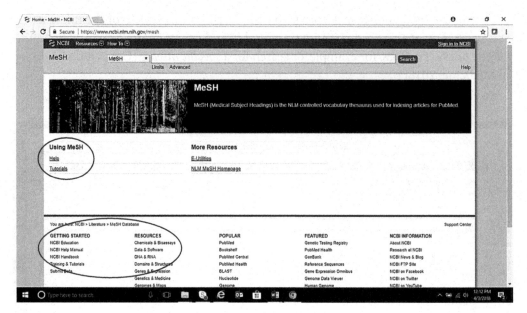

FIGURE 6.4

SOURCE: U.S. National Library of Medicine. (2018d). MeSH. An example of what you will see as you begin your search. Retrieved from https://www.ncbi.nlm.nih.gov/mesh.

For example, a search for myocardial infarction (the MeSH term for *heart attack*) will give you all the articles about heart attack regardless of whether the authors used the term *myocardial infarction* or *heart attack*. This is different from Internet search engines like Google that only search for the words entered (U.S. National Library of Medicine, 2018g).

Figure 6.5 shows another screen you may see as you search the literature. With this site you can search for *exact match* or terms or *fragments* of the search topic.

PubMed Health is another valuable site (Figure 6.6) where you can search for a full-text article alphabetically. You can see that with the letter A search 137 results were found. Be sure to explore the tabs across the top for even more information, for example, "Contents", "For researchers," and "What's New," and so on.

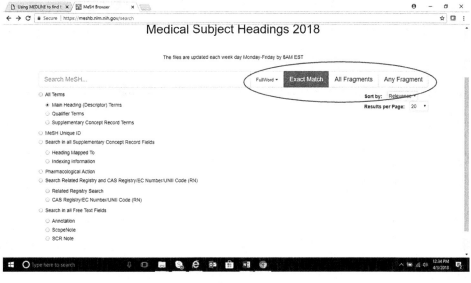

FIGURE 6.5

SOURCE: U.S. National Library of Medicine. (2018g). Search. Retrieved from https://meshb.nlm.nih.gov/search.

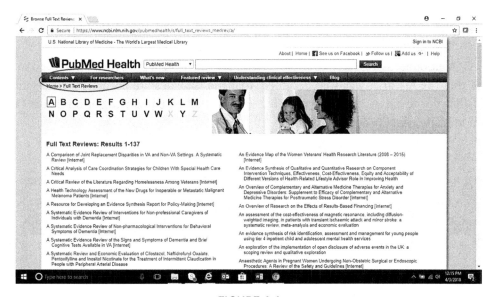

FIGURE 6.6

SOURCE: U.S. National Library of Medicine. (2018b). Full text reviews. Retrieved from https://www.ncbi.nlm.nih.gov/pubmedhealth/s/full_text_reviews_medrev.

MEDLINE (Figure 6.7) is a great resource to use for medical research because it is authoritative, peer reviewed, and complete (as much as possible, anyway). MEDLINE is authoritative because it permits you to see who exactly conducted the research, who wrote the results, and even where the research was conducted. The journals included in MEDLINE must target health professionals and researchers as their audience and publish original research.

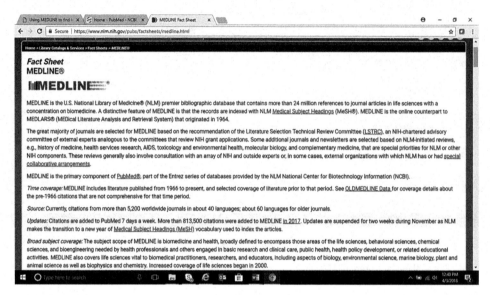

FIGURE 6.7

SOURCE: U.S. National Library of Medicine. (2018c). https://www.nlm.nih.gov/bsd/medline.html.

As mentioned, all research in MEDLINE is peer reviewed. Peer reviewers try to make sure that the research was well designed, that the statistics are accurately represented, and that the research is worthy of being shared, that is, convincing and reliable (U.S. National Library of Medicine, 2018a).

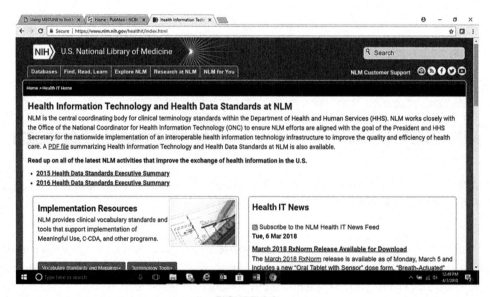

FIGURE 6.8

SOURCE: U.S. National Library of Medicine. (2018c). HealthIT. Retrieved from https://www.nlm.nih.gov/healthit/index.html.

The U.S. National Library of Medicine site (Figure 6.8) provides all of the most current up-to-date information on what's happening in the world of HealthIT, such as tools for meaningful use, terminology, *International Statistical Classification of Diseases*, 10th Revision (*ICD-10*) updates, and many other current, relevant topics that may impact clinical practice (U.S. National Library of Medicine, 2018c).

Critical Thinking Questions and Activities

- *As you read through the quantitative study in Exemplar 1, would you be able to conduct the study in the same way using smartphones?*
- *What other types of technology could you use to collect data?*
- *Select a topic of interest to you and go to the PubMed Health site to find a full-text article on that topic. What were the lessons learned as you stepped through this process?*
- *Find the YouTube tutorial on PubMed. Which site did you search to find it? Discuss what you learned from that tutorial.*
- *Which of the seven sites investigated here do you think will be most useful to your clinical practice?*

SUMMARY

This chapter introduced two categories of research for the BSN as well as any nurse interested in the basics of research—both qualitative and quantitative—as well as types of research; selected examples were provided.

Nursing research was defined and an explanation given as to why using research is important to nursing and clinical practice that links research and EBP using NI skills and technology to achieve better patient outcomes and safer and improved practice overall. Examples of healthcare areas that would impact practice were discussed.

The NINR agenda and its importance were introduced. The organization mandated that an NI research agenda continue through 2018 and be expanded to *all* users and challenged nurses to build on knowledge, guide the reengineering of nursing practice through the use of technology, and empower patients and their caregivers to engage in collaborative knowledge development, including the use of patient portals and other innovations.

Discussion of research challenges for the 2025 workforce were presented, as were increased technology use in e-Health and other areas of clinical practice. The importance of linking EBP and research using improved NI skill development was provided through the examples of how to perform electronic literature searches using selected sites and to find appropriate and relevant information to support EBP.

References

Abu-El-Noor, N. (2016). ICU nurses' perceptions and practice of spiritual care at the end of life: Implications for policy change. *OJIN: The Online Journal of Issues in Nursing, 21*(1). doi:10.3912/OJIN.Vol21No01PPT05

Agency for Healthcare Research and Quality. (2013). Funding & grants. Retrieved from www .ahrq.gov

American Association of Colleges of Nursing. (2008). *The essentials of baccalaureate education for professional nursing practice*. Washington, DC: Author. Retrieved from https://www .aacnnursing.org/Portals/42/Publications/BaccEssentials08.pdf

American Nurses Association. (2015). *Nursing informatics: Scope and standards of practice*. Silver Spring, MD: Author.

American Nurses Association. (2018). *What is nursing?* Retrieved from https://www .nursingworld.org/practice-policy/workforce/what-is-nursing

Association of College & Research Libraries (2014).Guidelines, Standards, and Frameworks, Retrieved From: www.ala.org/acrl/standards. March. p.1

Blake, N. (2016, April 29). Yes, nurses do research, and it's improving patient care. Elsevier Connect. Retrieved from https://www.elsevier.com

Canadian/American Spinal Research Organizations. (2015). Category: Research types. Retrieved from https://www.csro.com/portfolio/types-of-research

Cronenwett, L., Sherwood, G., Barnsteiner, J., Disch, J., Johnson, J., Mitchell, P., . . . Warren, J. (2007). Quality and Safety Education for Nurses. *Nursing Outlook, 55*(3), 122–131. doi:10.1016/j.outlook.2007.02.006

Cronenwett, L., Sherwood, G., Pohl, J., Barnsteiner, J., Moore, S., Sullivan, D., . . . Warren, J. (2009). Quality and safety education for advanced nursing practice. *Nursing Outlook 57*(6), 338–348.

Denzin, N. K., & Lincoln, Y. S. (2011). Editorial: Introductions to Parts 3 and 5. In N. K. Denzin & Y. S. Lincoln (Eds.), *Handbook of qualitative research* (4th ed., pp. 243–250, 563–568). Thousand Oaks, CA: Sage.

Despins, L. A., & Wakefield, B. J. (2018). The role of the electronic medical record in the intensive care unit nurse's detection of patient deterioration: a qualitative study. *CIN: Computers, Informatics, Nursing, 36*(6), 284–292. doi:10.1097/CIN.0000000000000431

Effken, J. (2003). An organizing framework for nursing informatics research. *Computers, Informatics, Nursing, 21*(6), 316–323; quiz 324–325.

Hunter, K.M. & Bickford, C.J. (2015). The practice specialty of nursing informatics. In V. K. Saba and K. A. McCormick (Eds.), *Essentials of nursing informatics* (6th ed., pp. 229–248). New York, NY: McGraw-Hill.

Institute of Medicine. (2015). Assessing progress on the IOM report: The future of nursing. Washington, DC: National Academies Press. Retrieved from https://www.nurse.com/ bog/2015/12/10/iom-releases-progress-report-on-future-of-nursing-2020-goals

Long, J. D., Gannaway, P., Ford, C., Doumit, R., Zeeni, N., Sukkarieh-Haraty, O., . . . Song, H. (2016). Effectiveness of a technology-based intervention to teach evidence-based practice: The EBR tool. *Worldviews on Evidence-Based Nursing, 13*(1), 59–65. doi:10.1111/wvn.12132

Malloy, D., Fahey-McCarthy, E., Murakami, M., Lee, Y., Choi, E., . . . Hadjistavropoulos, T. (2015). Finding meaning in the work of nursing: An international study. *OJIN: The Online Journal of Issues in Nursing, 20*(3). doi:10.3912/OJIN.Vol20No03PPT02

Medhanyie, A. A., Spigt, M., Yebyo, H., Little, A., Tadesse, K., . . . Blanco, R. (2017). Quality of routine health data collected by health workers using smartphone at primary health care in Ethiopia. *International Journal of Medical Informatics, 101*, 9–14. doi:10.1016/ j.ijmedinf.2017.01.016

Melnyk, B. M., Fineout-Overholt, E., Gallagher-Ford, L., & Kaplan, L. (2012). The state of evidence-based practice in US nurses: Critical implications for nurse leaders and educators. *JONA: The Journal of Nursing Administration, 42*(9), 410–417. doi:10.1097/ NNA.0b013e3182664e0a

Melnyk, B. M., Gallagher-Ford, L., Long, L. E., & Fineout-Overholt, E. (2014). The establishment of evidence-based practice competencies for practicing registered nurses and advanced practice nurses in real-world clinical settings: Proficiencies to improve healthcare quality, reliability, patient outcomes, and costs. *Worldviews on Evidence-Based Nursing, 11*(1), 5–15. doi:10.1111/wvn.12021

National Institute of Nursing Research. (2016). The NINR strategic plan: Advancing science, improving lives: A vision for nursing science. Retrieved from https://www.ninr.nih.gov/sites/files/docs/NINR_StratPlan2016_reduced.pdf

Newhouse, R., Barksdale, D. J., & Miller, J. A. (2015). The patient-centered outcomes research institute: research done differently. *Nursing Research, 64*(1), 72–77. doi:10.1097/NNR.0000000000000070

Oregon Health & Science University Library. (2018). What is EBP?—Evidence based practice toolkit for nursing. Retrieved from http://libguides.ohsu.edu/ebptoolkit

Patient-Centered Outcomes Research Institute. (2013). Mission and vision. Retrieved from www.pcori.org/research-results/patient-centered-outcomes-research

Quality and Safety Education for Nurses (QSEN). (2018). QSEN competencies. Retrieved from http://qsen.org/competencies/pre-licensure-ksas/#informatics

Risling, T. (2017). Educating the nurses of 2025: Technology trends of the next decade. *Nurse Education in Practice, 22*, 89–92. doi:10.1016/j.nepr.2016.12.007

Stevens, K. (2013). The impact of evidence-based practice in nursing and the next big ideas. *OJIN: The Online Journal of Issues in Nursing, 18*(2), Manuscript 4. doi:10.3912/OJIN.Vol18No02Man04

U.S. National Library of Medicine. (2018a). Fact sheet, MEDLINE. Retrieved from https://www.nlm.nih.gov/pubs/factsheets/medline.html

U.S. National Library of Medicine. (2018b). Full text reviews. Retrieved from https://www.ncbi.nlm.nih.gov/pubmedhealth/s/full_text_reviews_medrev

U.S. National Library of Medicine. (2018c). HealthIT. Retrieved from https://www.nlm.nih.gov/healthit/index.html

U.S. National Library of Medicine. (2018d). MeSH. Retrieved from https://www.ncbi.nlm.nih.gov/mesg

U.S. National Library of Medicine. (2018e). HealthIT. Retrieved from https://www.nlm.nih.gov/healthit/index.html

U.S. National Library of Medicine. (2018f). MeSH. Retrieved from https://www.ncbi.nlm.nih.gov/mesh

U.S. National Library of Medicine. (2018g). Search. Retrieved from https://meshb.nlm.nih.gov/search

World Health Organization. (1996). *International statistical classification of diseases*, tenth revision. Geneva, Switzerland: Author.

Yarcheski, A., & Mahon, N. E. (2013). Characteristics of quantitative nursing research from 1990 to 2010. *Journal of Nursing Scholarship, 45*(4), 405–411. doi:10.1111/jnu.12038

CHAPTER 7

NURSING INFORMATICS: APPLICATIONS TO SUPPORT EDUCATIONAL INITIATIVES

TARYN HILL | KAREN WEST

LEARNING OBJECTIVES AND OUTCOMES

Upon completion of this chapter, the reader will be able to:

- Describe the different learning environments and the roles they play in today's dynamic healthcare educational systems.

- Define current needed informatics skills to support information literacy and educational effectiveness in the baccalaureate-prepared nurse.

- Discuss the current and evolving roles of education in nursing informatics to support increased information management and application of patient care technology.

- Explore additional nursing informatics skills necessary for the baccalaureate-prepared nurse in today's healthcare setting.

☉ KEY NURSING INFORMATICS TERMS

Key concepts and terms you will hear in the discipline of nursing informatics are:

Computer knowledge

Computer literacy

Computer skills

Data collection

Data–information–knowledge–wisdom (DIKW)

Databases

Electronic health records (EHRs)

INTRODUCTION

As a practicing nurse you may already know that the most common technological interface used by nurses is the EHR. Previously, computerized systems were used in healthcare more as patient management systems rather than as systems used to collect, store, and analyze data. Patient management systems were used to check in and discharge patients, store data for billing information, and possibly had some administrative functions and limited functionality in the clinical area (ordering, lab, test, x-rays, and diets). The use of computers in nursing changed in part as a result of the drive to implement electronic documentation systems and to integrate other information systems within healthcare. Nurses were instructed in the use of the computer system that was used in their organization. Initial support was given prior to implementation of a different EHR system.

Consider what type of education you received in terms of navigating and using an EHR. Nurses mostly learned the basics of what was needed to manage workflow for their specific areas. Many EHR systems are a conglomerate of multiple programs integrated into one informational system. In some cases, the different programs do not communicate with each other, requiring nurses to access several different programs to find information on their patients. Consider how this may or may not impact patient care. Even nurses who are very tech-savvy became frustrated at the lack of interoperability found in these systems. To complete a task often took many steps; help desk personnel could only help with system functionality issues and nurses found themselves needing to use applications about which they had no education or exposure.

Changes in the electronic documentation system and programming came to them via in-house email notifications or as a continuing-education component that is assigned once a month. At times, this process left nurses feeling that after implementation of a new EHR, the nursing informatics (NI) team becomes an invisible entity in an office somewhere, increasing your workload but not sharing time to support nurses individually in their information system learning. Nurses learned things by memorizing the steps in a process, but many times did not stop to think about the "why" of the programs and how they use them as a nurse. Nurses should consider the fact that the EHR serves as a database and an informational tool to be used as a way to support their patients' care and to improve outcomes. The nurse should be the driver of this system instead of having the system define or drive the nurse's workflow.

Nursing informatics is defined as a discipline which supports nurses knowledge development using technology to support safe and effective nursing practice (Sipes et al., 2016). Consider what this definition means to you and how you would apply it in educational environments and the workplace.

▦ Question to Consider Before Reading On

1.   *What are some advantages to using technology in education?*

▦ Technology in Nursing Education

Technology changed the face, interaction, and rules of education through distance and online learning, which opened avenues for degree advancement that had never been seen before. The advent of online and distance learning provided a unique opportunity for individuals to begin a degree program that would complement their busy schedules.

This type of opportunity is possible through the advancements in technology that connected students electronically to higher education environments. These environments have blossomed, but the multitude of software programs needed to use these opportunities comes with an additional learning curve.

Learning the informatics skills needed to be able to use these different software programs can be directly correlated with NI skills. We first examine what you already know from working in the technologically enhanced healthcare work environment.

▦ Question to Consider Before Reading On

1.   *How do different educational environments support NI skills development?*

▦ Definitions

Information Literacy

This informatics skill supports nurses in educational environments as well as work environments. In this digital age, information is at everyone's fingertips, but how do you evaluate the quality of what you are reading? Consider all information with a discerning eye.

- ▦   What are the credentials of the author?
- ▦   Was the article peer reviewed? Is this information based on research or opinion?
- ▦   Where did you find it?

It is essential to determine the source of the information accessed online. For example, a wiki is an information resource that can be changed, usually by anyone who is logged in. Therefore, the information accessed through a wiki is not verified; an article found on a business website may be used to promote sales. However, a library system uses a validating process for the articles and research it includes. Healthcare-based information is usually found in large quantities in healthcare-focused journals and libraries.

Information Resources

Organizations have information resources they considered to be assets to the organization. These are the resources that assist in the use and management of data and information. In healthcare, these can be included in a library system or patient support system within an EHR and have been validated prior to inclusion. Some examples of specific programs that offer help to users are Micromedex for drug information and built-in computer-decision support systems, which are becoming more visible in support of evidence-based clinical care (Müller-Staub, de Graaf-Waar, & Paans, 2016).

Nurses use basic data analysis to look at vital sign trends, lab values, and additional output totals. Many EHRs can converge vital signs and other measures through menus that the nurse can access based on current patient needs. This type of submenu can assist nursing evaluation and can support decision processes in healthcare today. Consider what unique capabilities your EHR has. Analytics and quality improvement are processes that are defining change in healthcare (Strome, 2015). Nurses must understand the quality of data and how data are being used to change workflow and patient care processes within healthcare.

Quality Improvement

The concept of quality improvement refers to combined efforts of healthcare professionals to make changes within processes that will lead to better patient outcomes. It is a significant drive in healthcare today and is being supported by standards and benchmarking, which, in some cases, are tied to reimbursement (Darvish, Bahramnezhad, Keyhanian, & Navidhamidi, 2014). Nurses utilize informatics processes to meet patient needs. Nurses have a unique opportunity to be the maestro of the orchestra with regard to information systems they use at the point of care. Their collective voices can help improve processes because the point of care is a priority in improving quality and safety.

■ Questions to Consider Before Reading On

1. *What is VLE?*
2. *How is VLE accessed?*

■ Educational Environments Today

There are myriad learning environments that include the use of computer systems in nursing education and in healthcare. This variety of environments evolved from a technological idea that shaped ways to facilitate education. Educational venues in nursing include campus-based classrooms; hybrid systems that integrate both campus-based and online classes; online-only environments that allow students to complete coursework remotely; virtual learning environments (VLEs), including Second Life, which allow students to use their skills and competencies in pedagogy, group learning environments, and simulate face-to-face interaction in the VLE. Second Life is a free 3D virtual world online, where users can create, connect, and chat with others. Many universities use Second Life to give students an opportunity to explore real-world clinical scenarios in a safe environment.

Nursing also includes educational environments that use a computer for staff and patient learning. Patient health portals can also provide a learning environment for patients. Understanding the importance of NI competencies is an integral part of patient education and support of lifelong learning goals for nurses.

▓ Question to Consider Before Reading On

1. *How does NI competency and information literacy impact nursing education, patient care, and safety?*

▓ Nursing Informatics Skills and Learning Environments

Box 7.1 shows the different educational venues available in nursing today. The information in the box correlates computer and software programs the student will use in these educational environments and connects the needed NI skills for each type of learning system. This list is not all inclusive but lists some of the main software programs used today. Basic NI competencies are only listed under "campus based" but are applicable to each environment.

BOX 7.1

LEARNING ENVIRONMENTS, SOFTWARE PROGRAM INTERACTIONS, AND NI SKILLS NEEDE

EDUCATIONAL VENUE	COMPUTER INTERACTIONS	NI SKILLS
Campus based	Email Online registration Library resources Online file-sharing networks	Nursing knowledge (application of expertise and newly learned concepts) Computer skills Database utilization Information literacy Information management
Hybrid: Campus and online	Navigate learning management systems Submit assignments Library resources Email Online registration Online file sharing networks	Nursing knowledge (application of expertise and newly learned concepts) Computer skills Uploading files Microsoft Word proficiency Microsoft Excel proficiency Microsoft PowerPoint proficiency Virtual Meeting software proficiency
VLEs such as Second Life	Navigate in a virtual environment using an avatar	Nursing knowledge (application of expertise and newly learned concepts) Avatar interaction and movement in Second Life Virtual Meeting software proficiecny Uploading files

(continued)

BOX 7.1 (*continued*)

EDUCATIONAL VENUE	COMPUTER INTERACTIONS	NI SKILLS
Simulation, including Second Life	Low, mid, and high fidelity Computer-assisted simulation Onsite lab or virtual access	Nursing knowledge (application of expertise and newly learned concepts) Use of avatars in Second Life (virtual representation of a person used to interact with components of the learning environment) for role-playing, gestures, voice, can change clothes, use EHR and electronic medical records, has computer skills, is information literate (reviews best practices to develop a care plan), and is capabale of information management (data entry, can pull up past medical record information, can develop a graph with vital signs or intake and outputs and look at trends)
Staff learning environments	Online CPR modules Online continuing education Online competency assessments Online regulatory updates	Nursing knowledge (application of expertise and newly learned concepts) Access programming, enter responses, play videos, troubleshoot basic issues with lesson's download certificates, print out or send to our computer via email to save files
Patient learning environment	Hospital-based education for patients built into hospital information systems Able to find educational resources online	Nursing knowledge (application of expertise and newly learned concepts) Sharing electronic education with patients via hospital computer or tablet Computer skills Information literacy (find and confirm educational information quality before sharing; patient advocacy)
Patient portals	Computer-accessed platform that shares patient and physician information	Nursing knowledge Software programming and components: Learn by using these yourself, become skilled enocyte)

CPR, cardiopulmonary resuscitation; EHR, electronic health record; NI, nursing informatics; VLE, virtual learning environment.

Before starting a technology project, it is important to include a full self-assessment of the following competencies and skills:

- Computer skills
- Computer knowledge
- Information literacy
- Information management

The case scenario exemplars that follow focus on concepts to gain a better understanding of the models using DIKW theory.

CASE SCENARIO

EXEMPLAR 1

Brian has been studying the main concepts of NI, which include the need to understand and self-assess four key skills and competencies: computer skills, computer knowledge, information literacy, and information management. He starts to explore the different terminologies and decides to start with computer knowledge. He reviews information from the previous chapters on hardware and software terms.

Questions he explores are:

1. What is computer knowledge?
2. What does he need to know about the computer he will use?
3. What does he need to know about the operating system he will use?

Computer Knowledge: Basic, fundamental knowledge is necessary before engaging in a VLE.

1. Before you download Second Life, you must know what type of computer you are using. Are you using a PC or Mac?
2. You also need to know which operating system you are using.
3. You need to select the appropriate download based on your operating system. For Windows 10, see your system information using the following:
   a. Open the start menu.
   b. Perform a search for command prompt.
   c. Right click the result.
   d. Select "run as the administrator."
   e. Type the following command and press enter: system information
      https://www.google.com/searchq=how+to+find+out+the+operating
      +system+on+my+computer&rls=1C1CHWA_enUS620US621&oq
      =how+to+find+out+the+operating+sys&aqs=chrome.0.j69i57j0l4
      .11680j0j4&sourceid=chrome&ie=UTF-
4. You need to know whether you have a graphics card, the appropriate random access memory (RAM), and the central processing unit (CPU) necessary to support Second Life graphics to be able download the program.

(continued)

(continued)

EXEMPLAR 2

Brian continues to define, understand, and self-assess the next competency: computer skills. Again he reviews information from the previous chapters on hardware and software terms.

Questions he explores when searching for information include:

1. What are computer skills?
2. What type of activity would enhance and develop those skills?
3. Where are the classes to learn such skills?

Computer Skills: For each level of competency, the end user should understand both the types of programs being used and the special programs needed to accomplish goals. The student will be accessing a VLE (Second Life). Prebrief information will be given during class time. In the VLE, the student must complete the following computer skills:

1. Download Second Life to the computer.
2. Develop an account with a password.
3. Use the software to select an avatar.
4. Open course documents related to the assignment.
5. Use the email feature to correspond with the VLE staff and course instructor.
6. Upload or attach files to email and/or within the learning management system (LMS) to turn in assignment components.

Brian has completed both activities in Exemplars 1 and 2 as well as received good feedback from the class instructor that he is doing well in understanding and developing competency in these two areas.

▨ Questions to Consider Before Reading On

1. *What is your current knowledge deficit regarding NI and technology?*
2. *What is your professional responsibility in improving your NI competencies?*
3. *What impact would working in a VLE have on your NI competency development?*

▨ Understanding Nursing Informatics and Your Personal Nursing Informatics Knowledge Deficit

Use of technology in everyday life has expanded. This often leads to the misunderstanding that everyone in nursing today brings a high level of informatics knowledge and technology skill to the table (Williamson & Muckle, 2018). Many people learn things by memorization, but do not understand the theory or the knowledge behind what they do. For a nurse to be effective in a technology-inclusive work environment, she or he must understand the how, why, when, and where of technology to impact their practice and improve patient quality care (Strome, 2015). Many nurses struggle with using the software in front of them and lose sight of why they are using this program and how this technology helps in patient care.

In higher education, students are exposed to and are expected to have or learn the basic computer skills considered necessary to complete their coursework. In an effort to make the technology used meaningful to nursing students, information and/or practice with this technology has been included in curricula development. "Course work and clinical experiences will expose graduates to a range of technologies that facilitate clinical care, including patient monitoring systems, medication administration systems, and other technologies to support patient care" (American Association of Colleges of Nursing [AACN], 2008, p. 18).

One way for a nurse to evaluate her or his skills to better understand whether she or he has a personal NI knowledge deficit is to take a competency survey. A competency survey will allow the nurse to self-assess basic informatics skills using a tool that will assist in identifying areas that can strengthen their knowledge and skills (Choi & Bakken, 2013). Several tools are available and are being used in nursing education environments, but have not been made available for the working nurse. A tool known as the *TIGER-Based Assessment of Nursing Informatics Competencies* (*TANIC*) can be used by the nurse to assess their individual competency level (Hunter, McGonigle, & Hebda, 2013). You can see competencies from this tool in Box 7.3. We recommend that you use TANIC to assess your own competency level and reflect on your results.

NI skills are much more than just program and computer skills. They involve understanding electronic health systems and being able to capitalize on information resources, patient data and evidence-based practice knowledge and to use that information to support safety and better patient outcomes. Every nurse must understand the NI theory of DIKW and how it applies to nursing (Ronquillo, Currie, & Rodney, 2016). You were introduced to DIKW theory in Chapter 2. Box 7.2 shows the application of this theory to a nursing patient scenario in an educational environment in which DIKW is applied.

BOX 7.2

COMPARISON OF NURSING PROCESS, NURSING INFORMATICS THEORY, AND BASIC EXAMPLES?

NURSING PROCESS	DIKW IN NURSING ENVIRONMENT	EDUCATION ENVIRONMENT EXAMPLE OF DIKW
Assessment	Data and information (data are raw facts). Temperature, pulse, respiration, and blood pressure, each of these is data. It becomes information when it is placed into a format that supports evaluation against criteria. One set of vital signs can give you an idea whether a patient is within medical norms.	**Data**: individual characters—1, 2, 3, a, d, z . . . **Information**: Data is placed into a format that enhances definition, understanding, or learning Student Guide for virtual learning environment
	EHR at the bedside—you can enter the form for vital signs and look at a 24-hour list of vital signs, then a 480 hour and 72-hours list or you can use a program feature and change these vital signs into a graph that shows peaks and trends.	**I. Interacting with objects in the virtual learning environment** You interact with objects in the virtual learning environment by using the cursor on your mouse and through avatar use.
Diagnosis	Knowledge (i.e., applying your nursing knowledge and ability in combination with medical information specific to this patient). Patient has COPD and is admitted with pneumonia (found in the physician admission assessment and patient history on the computer at the patient bedside). Your nursing knowledge that COPD traps air and makes oxygen exchange difficult and can lead to full respiratory arrest if not treated, is essential to patient care.	Course assignment that must be completed using technology Student's technology objective is to meet assignment goals. *I need to be able to use my computer and interact with different things in the VLE.*

(continued)

BOX 7.2 (*continued*)

NURSING PROCESS	DIKW IN NURSING ENVIRONMENT	EDUCATION ENVIRONMENT EXAMPLE OF DIKW
Outcome planning	Knowledge and wisdom "Your oxygen is on and working; you have a fever, which is making it harder to breathe. I will work to get your fever down." "I have called the respiratory therapist and she will help us make your breathing better. I am here and will be taking care of you until you are feeling better."	Taking **information** and adding **knowledge,** personal, course supplied, or gained through individual research **II. Student self-assessment of technology and skills needed to complete the assignment** 1. Do I know how to use my mouse in the VLE? 2. Do I know how to get an avatar and be able to move it around with my computer? 3. Is there an orientation for this? 4. Is support available support if I have a problem? Technology programs to use: 1. Microsoft Windows 10 2. Computer is 2 years old so I think it will work 3. I have a mouse connected to my computer
		4. I can use a Microsoft Word document to guide me through the assignment and can use same document to complete a course assignment. 5. I use email communication with my teacher as well as use it to turn in my assignment. 6. I have Internet access that is effective in my online course so i hope it will be effective in this learning environment. **III. Student professional knowledge** 1. Student has worked as an associate degree nurse in an emergency room. 2. Student understands the riage system as used in the ER. 3. Student has had some disaster training through continuing education required for his ER position. 4. Student has CPR certification. 5. Student researched disaster triage and the community health nurse's role in cases of disaster.

(continued)

BOX 7.2 (*continued*)

NURSING PROCESS	DIKW IN NURSING ENVIRONMENT	EDUCATION ENVIRONMENT EXAMPLE OF DIKW
Implementation	Nursing skill and knowledge/ technology knowledge and application	**Information** and **knowledge** needed to do the assignment: Course assignment includes using an avatar to create a disaster scenario, triage multiple patients in the field, acting as a community health nurse. 1. Read all material given for the assignment. 2. Downloaded Second Life successfully. 3. Chose an avatar. 4. Went through orientation to learn how to interact using the avatar. 5. Followed directions to get to assignment area. 6. Completed the assignment. 7. Attached completed form to email. 8. Sent email to course instructor.
Evaluation	Assessment, outcomes of (document all applicable data, which will become Information for healthcare team)	**Knowledge to wisdom** Student will evaluate the course assignment. Student will identify and respond to course objectives for this assignment. **Wisdom** 1. Student will take the technology knowledge learned during preparation of this assignment and use it in the technology-driven world of nursing. 2. Students will gain knowledge of a community health nurse role in a disaster and understand the importance of disaster training. 3. Understand how education through simulation and scenario support can support educational objectives.

COPD, chronic obstructive pulmonary disease; DIKW, data–information–knowledge–wisdom; EHR, electronic health record; ER, emergency room.

CASE SCENARIO (CONTINUED)
EXEMPLAR 3

Brian continues to define, understand, and self-assess the next competency—information literacy. Again he reviews information from the previous chapters on hardware and software terminology and is taking a course in which he learned about the concept of DIKW.

The questions Brian reviews include:

1. What information do I need in order to complete this assignment?
2. Where can I search to find the information I need?

Information Literacy: It is important to know where to go to identify and validate the information you need.

1. Review the course material related to the assignment.
2. Download from https://secondlife.com/support/downloads
3. Complete the two searches in Exemplar 1 to identify the valuable information needed about your computer to be able to run the program.

Brian reviews the steps and activities listed in Box 7.2 and completes a self-assessment to define what information he needs.

EXEMPLAR 4

Brian continues to define, understand, and self-assess the next competency—information management. Again he reviews information from the previous chapters on hardware and software terms and is taking a course in which he has learned about the concept of DIKW, as described earlier.

Questions Brian reviews include:

1. Was the activity accurately completed?
2. Did I have the appropriate skill and competency needed to complete the assignments?
3. What do I need to work on to further develop my weakest skill?

Information Management: This occurs when you have applied what you have learned to accomplish the tasks needed to complete your assignment. Information management is an NI skill that involves thinking processes. These include your knowledge of the subject matter and how you use technological knowledge and skills to meet your goals and objectives.

1. Read and download the proper course information related to the assignment.
2. Read and follow other information that is given to you by your VLE staff mentors.

(continued)

(continued)

Reflecting on these exemplars, read the questions posed here and work through the activities suggested. What questions would you still want to explore with your faculty or VLE staff mentors?

1. What would you take from this to apply to your practice?
2. What suggestions would you have to enhance the VLE for future students?

The screenshot shown in Figure 7.1 depicts what your computer screen might look like if you have a number of applications loaded onto it.

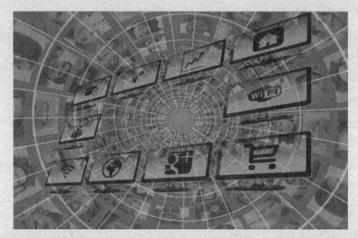

FIGURE 7.1 This what your computer screen might look like. Note the possibilities.

SOURCE: https://pixabay.com/en/monitor-computer-screen-hardware-862135.

▓ Questions to Consider Before Reading On

1. *What is your priority learning need related to current technology?*
2. *Were you surprised by the results of your TANIC self-assessment?*
3. *How will you maximize newly learned skills to improve the DIKW process in your work?*

▓ Plan Development to Define Needs of Users in Application to Nursing Informatics

Nurses

All nurses need NI competencies to be effective in their technology-driven work. Fortunately, most computer programming has a similar format. The EHR system you use

1. Basic computer skills: Asses your skills using the TANIC.
2. Assess the areas in which you need to increase your computer knowledge and skills.
3. Develop a plan to acquire this additional proficiency.
4. Examine your proficiencies related to:
   a. Microsoft Windows
   b. Microsoft Word
   c. Microsoft Excel
   d. Microsoft Outlook
   e. Microsoft PowerPoint
   f. Microsoft Publisher

at work may have multiple menus and functionality, which could be similar to those you use in other programs. Spend some time looking at these menus.

Many menus and functionality found in these programs are also used in other software programs. Microsoft offers free education for each of its applications. Take some time to consider the changes and updates that have occurred among different versions of Microsoft products and your current competency. Identify whether the functionality has changed over time (González, Schachner, Tattone, & Benítez, 2016). Familiarizing yourself with the functionalities of these programs can support your use of NI competencies. Increasing your computer competencies will help you to stop struggling with the programming and start thinking about why this software or program is available. Consider how you can utilize this technology to improve nursing knowledge and practice as well as increase quality and safety for patients.

Patient

Patients also come to the healthcare arena with various levels of informatics skills and knowledge. Technology has become a constant in healthcare and it is important that nurses support their own skill and knowledge to be able to teach their healthcare consumers. The patient's connection to the healthcare arena is a nurse the majority of the time. "A growing number of 'health citizens' and 'e-patients' (empowered, engaged, equipped, and enabled) are deepening their participation in their own health care through personal health-information tools" (Hull, 2015, para. 3).

It is the nurses' responsibility to support patient education and safety with the technology they are using as well as the technology that they need to learn to be able to support patients' individual health needs. Patients have difficulty using patient portals, and some type of orientation or education component is recommended to increase their abilities in using this technology (Kruse, Argueta, Lopez, & Nair, 2015). EHRs, social media sights, appropriate medication-information sites, and online appointment processes are just a few of the areas that patients are using to support their healthcare. Nurses need to assess their patients' and families educational deficits related to the technology they are using and work toward decreasing these with every encounter (Box 7.3).

BOX 7.3

TECHNOLOGY AND SUBJECT KNOWLEDGE SELF-ASSESSMENT SCALE (BASED ON THE TANIC TOOL)

The following is a self-assessment scale that assists the individual in looking at the three prebrief or preassessment areas necessary to develop a technology and subject knowledge self-assessment to guide preparation for a project or educational offering in our technology-driven world.

TECHNOLOGY AND SUBJECT KNOWLEDGE SELF-ASSESSMENT SCALE	POOR	FAIR	GOOD	VERY GOOD	EXCELLENT
Personal/professional knowledge of subject	1—No exposure or knowledge of subject	2—Some exposure or knowledge (I know what that is.)	3—Knows about the subject and understands primary usage	4—Able to define subject without research; able to identify multiple uses	5—Understands subject; is proficient and can apply in any situation
Computer skills (Laptop and/or desktop keyboard skills)	1—Doesn't know how to turn on computer or laptop Doesn't know how to check for Internet connection	2—Can turn on device; uses keyboard with correct fingers; knows how to check on Internet access and create a connection	3—Not just surfing on the "Net"; uses keyboard shortcuts Ctrl-C = copy Can use Control-Alt-Delete to stop a program that has locked up the computer	4—Knows F-key functionalities Initial F-key functionalities: F1 usually opens a help menu F3 can open a search window on the Windows desktop F3 on an Apple computer running MacOS can open Mission Control program (Computer Hope, 2018)	5—Understands how to use all keys on the keyboard and knows to check for special functionality in different programming

Software programming needed to accomplish task (Microsoft Word/Microsoft Excel, Access, specific software programs used for project or educational opportunity)	1—Does not understand that Microsoft Word and Microsoft Excel are different software programs designed for different tasks	2—Understands that each different program has a unique programming purpose	3—Able to apply knowledge of what a program does to effectively complete a project	4—Understands enough about what different programs do to search for and utilize a program not basic to their computer	5—Can utilize multiple different types of software programs to meet goals and complete projects

You do not need to be an expert in the subject matter or technology being utilized for your project or educational endeavor. Preplanning with some initial research will assist you with basic knowledge of your subject area (a field to grow on) and decrease your frustration related to the programming you need to use to accomplish your goal. (If you scored below a 3 in any area of this process, then you need to do initial research on those areas related to your project.)

■ Questions to Consider Before Reading On

1. *How can the technology you are using help you with your patient care?*

2. *Is there any part of the information system that you are utilizing that can help improve patient quality?*

3. *Does your EHR have a library or resource that you can access to help with use of the applications or software updates to fill in any gaps in your knowledge? Can you develop a plan on how to evaluate your level of NI competency?*

4. *Do you know how to develop a personal health record and how to validate health information sources on the Internet?*

5. *Can you teach patients how to validate health information sources on the Internet?*

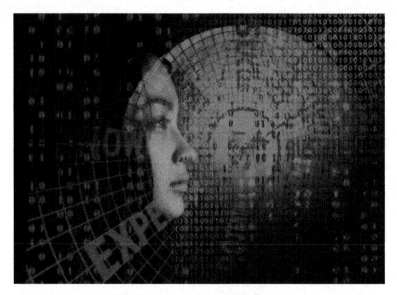

FIGURE 7.2 Technology of the future.

SOURCE: https://pixabay.com/en/technology-abstract-data-3093707.

■ Future Technology

Continuing education has become a significant part of nursing in the 21st century. Education will continue to become more virtual and likely will use augmented reality to look at "real-time" active learning and evaluation. *E-learning* is a term used for education that is accessed electronically. E-learning has been implemented for nurses in higher education environments, continuing education in work environments, and has been developed for patient education as well.

Technology information and its use in healthcare is a concept that continues to expand. Future directions include mobile health; telehealth; robotics; and sensors that can continuously monitor blood pressure, blood glucose levels, oxygen levels, ECG, and weight monitoring (Majumder et al., 2017). In order for this type of technology to be effective it will need to be accessible to everyone. In addition, there will be a need for data to be imported into a healthcare record or documentation system that includes information supporting decisions made by healthcare practitioners.

Data from any source must be accessible, savable, and able to be incorporated into a pertinent documentation system. Nurses will import or export data from these types of programs in order to manage patient care outcomes. Therefore, they need to understand communication technology, encryption, and decryption to be able to protect personal health records and to access and import information (downloading). The nurse at the point of care should be the person who will access a patient's Fitbit or other monitoring device, for example; he or she has to download the data for review of vital signs and heart rhythm patterns over time for continued collaborative patient healthcare management.

The use of advanced technology to manage patient symptoms will help to determine the plan of care and desired outcome for the patient (U.S. Department of Health and Human Services [HHS], 2018). Examples of advanced augmented technology include STATworkUP and Symptom Mate. These are mobile health applications designed to support providers with useful tools used to assist with interventions and to support knowledge needed to manage patients. These types of applications are designed to assist in collecting patient data that can help determine plans of care that will be most efficient and yield the best results.

Quality and safety in nursing will be directly affected by nurse's knowledge about modern technology being used and understanding how to use it effectively. Technology can be imperfect, and it will need nursing judgment to be used safely. Smart pumps have incorporated some safety skills into infusion management. Smart pumps have been loaded with medication directories that include safe rates of administration and safe strengths for medications with elevated risks. These make it easier for the nurse to verify and check the pump settings against the patient orders.

- Is the in-house pharmacy medication mixture and infusion rate available in the directory?
- Can you manually change the mixture and infusion rate (with second-nurse verification) to comply with physician orders?
- If you do a manual change, will the EHR import this documentation effectively?

Remember that information was entered by other people to develop these infusion modules. It is important to double-check the infusion rate, time of administration, and strength by what is ordered and what you know. Technology is not infallible, and the nurse is the last checkpoint for safety. Find out what you need to know about the technology that will affect the patients in your care. If technology is introduced that you are unfamiliar with, request formal education for yourself and your peers.

Educational environments in nursing are here to support nurses' acquisition of nursing theory, nursing knowledge, and skills to be safe and effective practitioners of healthcare. No matter which type of educational environment you are using, NI will be included. NI skills are a combination of nursing knowledge, computer skills, information literacy, and information management. Embrace all of the experiences developed for you and keep an inquiring mind about the technology used now and to be developed in the future. An effective nurse is a nurse who can use NI to support practice and decision-making, thereby supporting quality and safety in healthcare. At the center of everything is the need for the baccalaureate-prepared nurse to participate in evaluating different information systems across our healthcare practice settings and support changes and enhancements to policy and procedure development.

Your nursing knowledge added to your work experience and knowledge of electronic-driven information systems makes you a central and important player supporting change of current systems to make them more effective in the work and/or educational environment. Feedback, questions, and suggestions for improvements are important to support patient safety and future nursing education.

QSEN SCENARIO

An RN from the previous shift has left a report on one of your patients. The nurse stated that the medication administration bar-code reader was not working properly throughout the shift. The nurse did not contact the IT department, but instead used an override code to provide medications to the patient. When you assess the patient, you discover that the incorrect intravenous (IV) solution is being administered.

- What action is your priority?
- What are the appropriate steps in managing this scenario?
- What gaps in NI competencies occurred during the previous shift?
- How would you have handled the situation?
- What follow-up is needed?

▮ Questions to Consider Before Reading On

1. *What are some ways NI and patient safety are linked?*
2. *Consider how you can best continue to develop your knowledge base using NI to support quality and patient care. What are some activities you will be involved in to accomplish this?*
3. *What are four roles a BSN with NI knowledge and skills can assume?*
4. *What national organizations' mandates have impacted the need for increasing NI competencies in healthcare?*

▮ Applications of Nursing Informatics: DIKW

You have had an opportunity to explore and self-assess basic skills, knowledge, and competencies in the scenarios and activities provided. As you review the AACN Essentials listed in Box 7.4, consider how you can best continue to develop your knowledge base using NI to support quality and patient care. What are some activities you will be involved in to accomplish this? Can you accomplish all of the skills and activities listed? If not what, will you do to develop that skill, knowledge, and competency?

BOX 7.4

AACN ESSENTIALS APPLICABLE TO NURSING INFORMATICS
AACN ESSENTIAL IV

1. Demonstrate skills in using patient care technologies, information systems, and communication devices that support safe nursing practice.
2. Use telecommunication technologies to assist in effective communication in a variety of healthcare settings.
3. Apply safeguards and decision-making support tools embedded in patient care technologies and information systems to support a safe practice environment for both patients and healthcare workers.
4. Understand the use of CIS systems to document interventions related to achieving nurse-sensitive outcomes.
5. Use standardized terminology in a care environment that reflects nursing's unique contribution to patient outcomes.
6. Evaluate data from all relevant sources, including technology, to inform the delivery of care.
7. Recognize the role of information technology in improving patient care outcomes and creating a safe care environment.
8. Uphold ethical standards related to data security, regulatory requirements, confidentiality, and clients' right to privacy.
9. Apply patient care technologies as appropriate to address the needs of a diverse patient population.
10. Advocate for the use of new patient care technologies for safe, quality care.
11. Recognize that redesign of workflow and care processes should precede implementation of care technology to facilitate nursing practice.
12. Participate in evaluation of information systems in practice settings through policy and procedure development.

SOURCE: American Association of Colleges of Nursing. (2008). *Executive summary: The essentials of baccalaureate education for professional nursing practice. Essential IV: Information management and application of patient care technology* (pp. 18–19). Washington, DC: Author. Retrieved from http://www.aacnnursing.org/Portals/42/Publications/BaccEssentials08.pdf.

(continued)

BOX 7.4 (*continued*)

AACN MASTER'S ESSENTIAL V

1. Analyze current and emerging technologies to support safe practice environments and to optimize patient safety, cost-effectiveness, and health outcomes.
2. Evaluate outcome data using current communication technologies, information systems, and statistical principles to develop strategies to reduce risks and improve health outcomes.
3. Promote policies that incorporate ethical principles and standards for the use of health and information technologies.
4. Provide oversight and guidance in the integration of technologies to document patient care and improve patient outcomes.
5. Use information and communication technologies, resources, and principles of learning to teach patients and others.
6. Use current and emerging technologies in the care environment to support lifelong learning for self and others.

SOURCE: American Association of Colleges of Nursing. (2011). *The Essentials of master's education in nursing. Essential V: Informatics and healthcare technologies* (p. 19). Washington, DC: Author. Retrieved from http://www.aacnnursing.org/Portals/42/Publications/MastersEssentials11.pdf.

■ Critical Thinking Questions and Activities

Now that you have had an opportunity to reflect on and review the activities and scenarios in this chapter, considering your strengths in basic computer skills, what was the outcome of the self-assessment of skills you completed?

- *What areas are most important for you to develop?*
- *How will development of these areas assist you in practice?*
- *What relevance will they have to improving quality and safety in patient care?*
- *How can you be a catalyst in your practice area for improving overall NI competencies?*
- *In what way can you help to enhance the health literacy of your patients?*

SUMMARY

Educational environments today work to include NI skills by supporting the three major components of NI: computer skills, informatics skills, and information literacy. Increasing awareness of nurse's current knowledge, information management skills, and individual technology deficits related to current and future work environments prepares nursing for future change. Continued learning is the most effective when it is individually driven.

Nursing students need to identify their technology knowledge deficits and become familiar with the NI skills and knowledge they so possess. Utilizing self-assessment tools is a great way for individual nurses to support their educational needs. Once a knowledge deficit has been identified, it is important to develop a plan of action to improve on this knowledge. Following through a plan of action supports individual strengths and creates a stronger nursing workforce. Nursing students need to embrace every opportunity to use technology to support education using outside research and skills practice in order to support and facilitate increased quality and safety in healthcare.

References

American Association of Colleges of Nursing. (2008). *Executive summary: The essentials of baccalaureate education for professional nursing practice. Essential IV: Information management and application of patient care technology* (pp. 18–19). Washington, DC: Author. Retrieved from http://www.aacnnursing.org/Portals/42/Publications/BaccEssentials08.pdf

American Association of Colleges of Nursing. (2011). *The essentials of master's education in nursing. Essential V: Informatics and healthcare technologies* (p. 19). Washington, DC: Author. Retrieved from http://www.aacnnursing.org/Portals/42/Publications/MastersEssentials11.pdf

Choi, J., & Bakken, S. (2013). Validation of the Self-assessment of Nursing Informatics Competencies Scale among undergraduate and graduate nursing students. *Journal of Nursing Education, 52*(5), 257–282. doi:10.3928/01484834-20130412-01

Computer Hope. (2018). Computer keyboard shortcut keys. Retrieved from https://www .computerhope.com/shortcut.htm

Darvish, A., Bahramnezhad, F., Keyhanian, S., & Navidhamidi, M. (2014). The role of nursing informatics on promoting quality of health care and the need for appropriate education. *Global Journal of Health Science, 6*(6), 11–18. doi:10.5539/gjhs.v6n6p11

González, Z. A., Schachner, M. B., Tattone, M. A., & Benítez, S. E. (2016). Changing educational paths in an informatics course according to the needs and expectations of nursing degree students. *Studies in Health Technology and Informatics, 225*, 324–328.

Hull, S. (2015). Using technology to engage patients. *American Nurse Today, 10*(9), 1.

Hunter, K., McGonigle, D., & Hebda, T. (2013). TIGER-based measurement of nursing informatics competencies: The development and implementation of an online tool for self-assessment. *Journal of Nursing Education and Practice (JNEP), 3*(12), 70–80. doi:10.5430/jnep.v3n12p70

Kruse, S. C., Argueta, D. A., Lopez, L., & Nair, A. (2015). Patient and provider attitudes toward the use of patient portals for the management of chronic disease: A systematic review. *Journal of Medical Internet Research, 17*(2), 16. doi:10.2196/jmir.3703

Majumder, S., Aghayi, E., Noferesti, M., Memarzadeh-Tehran, H., Mondal, T., . . . Deen, M. (2017). Smart homes for elderly healthcare—Recent advances and research challenges. *Sensors, 17*(11), 2496. doi:10.3390/s17112496

Müller-Staub, M., de Graaf-Waar, H., & Paans, W. (2016). An internationally consented standard for nursing process-clinical decision support systems in electronic health records. *Computers, Informatics, Nursing: CIN, 34*(11), 493–502. doi:10.1097/CIN.0000000000000277

Ronquillo, C., Currie, L., & Rodney, P. (2016). The evolution of data–information-knowledge -wisdom in nursing informatics. *Advances in Nursing Science, 39*(1), 1–18. doi:10.1097/ans.0000000000000107

Sipes, C., McGonigle, D., Hunter, K., Hebda, T., Hill, T., & Lamblin, J. (2016). Operationalizing the TANIC and NICA-L3/L4 tools to improve informatics competencies. *Studies in Health Technology and Informatics, 225,* 292–296.

Strome, T. (2015). Why nurses must understand analytics and quality improvement. Retrieved from http://healthcareanalytics.info/2015/04/why-nurses-must-understand-analytics-and-quality-improvement/#.WvCBDYgvyUk

U.S. Department of Health and Human Services. (2018). Mobile medical apps. Retrieved from https://www.fda.gov/MedicalDevices/DigitalHealth/MobileMedicalApplications/default.htm#a

Williamson, K. M., & Muckle, J. (2018). Students' perception of technology use in nursing education. *CIN: Computers, Informatics, Nursing, 36*(2), 70. doi:10.1097/CIN.0000000000000396

PART IV

NURSING INFORMATICS: DATA APPLICATIONS

CHAPTER 8

DATA STANDARDIZATION APPLICATIONS—CAPTURING DATA

LISA M. BLAIR | LYNDA HARDY

LEARNING OBJECTIVES AND OUTCOMES

Upon completion of this chapter, the reader will be able to:

- Define data standardization.
- Discuss the rationale for standardizing nursing-generated data.
- Discuss the differences and applications for three standardized nursing nomenclatures.
- List two references for data standardization.
- Identify two outcomes of data standardization.

☉ KEY NURSING INFORMATICS TERMS

Some of the key concepts and terms you will hear in this chapter are:

Agency for Healthcare Research and Quality (AHRQ)

Common Data Model

Data standardization

Data harmonization

Electronic health record (EHR)

Evidence-based practice

Logical Observation Identifiers Names and Codes (LOINC)

Machine readable

Nursing Interventions Classification (NIC)

◉ **KEY NURSING INFORMATICS TERMS** (*continued*)

Nursing Minimum Data Set (NMDS)

Nursing Outcomes Classification (NOC)

National Quality Measures Clearinghouse (NQMC)

Patient-Reported Outcomes Measurement Information System (PROMIS)

Systemized Nomenclature of Medicine (SNOMED)

INTRODUCTION

You already know and understand that documentation practices may vary depending on work environment, formal and informal educational background, and personal interest in technology. Some nurses may have limited exposure to technology, while others may interact with data generated by electronic health records (EHRs), insulin pumps, patient wearables, other devices (e.g., glucometer), or imaging and lab report visualization. The intensive care environment offers a vast array of data generated by patient monitors, electronic pumps, ventilators, and other equipment that nurses may be required to document or validate. In each of these cases, patient data must be easily accessed and understandable to all members of the care team. The process of ensuring that data are accessible, understandable, and usable by multiple people are steps in data standardization.

▓ Questions to Consider Before Reading On

1. *How do patient data differ based on the practice setting where it is created?*

2. *What kinds of technology are in use in your practice environment that might contribute rich data to the patient record?*

CASE SCENARIO—JOHN AND Mrs. BAKER

John is an associate's degree–prepared registered nurse providing care for Mrs. Baker after knee replacement surgery. He prepares a routine medication for administration at 9 a.m. by scanning his ID and entering a code into the dispensary machine to get the medication. When arriving in the patient's room he notices that Mrs. Baker looks uncomfortable and seems restless. He asks Mrs. Baker to verify her name and identification information as he uses the bedside computer to scan her wrist band and double-check the medication order.

He asks Mrs. Baker how she is feeling as he opens the medication and passes her a cup of water. Mrs. Baker reports feeling ok but says her pain has been worsening in the last hour and that she would like a pain pill. John assesses Mrs. Baker's pain and documents his assessment and the routine medication he administered in her EHR. He reviews what he needs to do next:

(*continued*)

(continued)

1. What data has John collected and documented about Mrs. Baker?
2. Who else might need this data? How might it be used to improve her care?
3. What other members of the healthcare team entered documentation about Mrs. Baker?
4. How might the accessibility or lack thereof of this information affect John's work?

▨ Questions to Consider Before Reading On

1. *What are three functions supported by data standardization?*
2. *What issues can be resolved with data standardization when using checklists versus free text?*
3. *What are the benefits of data standardization?*

▨ What Is Data Standardization and Why Does It Matter?

The term "data standardization" is not unique to healthcare. IBM (2015) defines data standardization as "the process by which similar data received in various formats is transformed to a common format that enhances the comparison process." Observational Health Data Sciences and Informatics (2018) defines data standardization as a critical process of creating or assuring that patient data are available, understandable, and usable for functions that are important to the patient, nursing, and society.

The EHR was created in a physician-centric manner. Physician notes are often "automatic," meaning that as a physician begins to type in a patient-related note, the EHR is programmed to understand the context within which the note is being written and often completes the note. This information, having been programmed into the system, is *machine readable* (Box 8.1).

BOX 8.1

FUNCTIONS SUPPORTED BY DATA STANDARDIZATION

- ▨ Public health and safety monitoring
- ▨ Medical and nursing research
- ▨ Insurance and Medicaid/Medicare reimbursement
- ▨ Staff scheduling and acuity determinations
- ▨ Direct patient care
- ▨ Trend analysis
- ▨ Quality improvement

SOURCE: Reprint Courtesy of International Business Machines Corporation, © International Business Machines Corporation.

The use of machine-readable documentation has several benefits. Physicians benefit by having reduced documentation time from auto-fill and other functions, making documenting easier. Nurses, other healthcare team members, and patients benefit from having consistent and legible documentation of physician findings and orders formatted for rapid identification of specific information. Beyond the bedside, managers, billing departments, and accreditation entities benefit by being able to rely on the computer to accurately and quickly code physician data for a range of legal, business, and financial purposes. And in research and quality improvement efforts, machine-readable physician documentation makes prescreening for participants and abstracting data from the medical record considerably less time consuming and challenging than past efforts using paper records or non–machine-readable documentation.

Consider how you, as a nurse, document patient signs, symptoms, and problems. Some EHR systems have check boxes for signs or symptoms, while others use free text. The issue is nursing notes may not be machine readable. When words, notes, numbers, and characters are machine readable, they are able to be automatically processed by a computer. Automatic processing allows data to become information that can be trended and applied to patient care and beyond.

CASE SCENARIO (CONTINUED)

John reviews Mrs. Baker's medication record and sees that she has not had pain medication for 6 hours. Her surgeon has ordered pain medication q4h, PRN, and the order has been verified by a pharmacist. John returns to the dispensary, selects the appropriate medication from the patient available list, and prepares the medication for delivery. After verifying identity and giving her the medication, John helps Mrs. Baker reposition in bed and makes sure she has access to water and call light.

He documents the medication delivery and goes to answer a call light from another patient. About an hour later, John returns to check on Mrs. Baker, who reports her pain has decreased to a tolerable level. John documents Mrs. Baker's pain reassessment in the EHR. He reflects:

1. How would documenting the pain assessment and medication administration in a system without *machine readability* alter Mrs. Baker's care and outcomes?

2. How might Mrs. Baker's documentation be used when nurses on the unit decide to undertake a project to see if an evidence-based practice change to postoperative pain management is needed?

▓ Question to Consider Before Reading On

1. *What are three main areas and departments that are affected when data are not machine-readable?*

Improving Processes and Outcomes Through Standardization

How nurses document patient assessments, education, and outcomes has an impact on patient care. Lack of machine-readable documentation can result in inefficiencies and safety problems in direct patient care, but consider how other uses of data might be affected by lack of machine readability. Consider what might happen if John fails to document Mrs. Baker's care in the standardized manner in the EHR (Box 8.2).

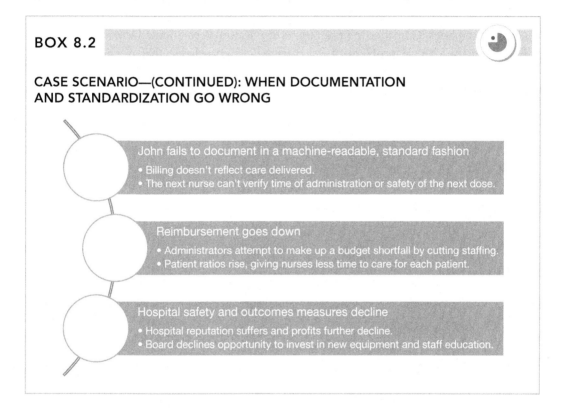

BOX 8.2

CASE SCENARIO—(CONTINUED): WHEN DOCUMENTATION AND STANDARDIZATION GO WRONG

John fails to document in a machine-readable, standard fashion
- Billing doesn't reflect care delivered.
- The next nurse can't verify time of administration or safety of the next dose.

Reimbursement goes down
- Administrators attempt to make up a budget shortfall by cutting staffing.
- Patient ratios rise, giving nurses less time to care for each patient.

Hospital safety and outcomes measures decline
- Hospital reputation suffers and profits further decline.
- Board declines opportunity to invest in new equipment and staff education.

▧ Question to Consider Before Reading On

1.   Define CDE. How do CDEs support data quality?

Standardization of healthcare terms has been placed into context by the use of *common data elements* (CDEs). CDEs are defined as "variables that are operationalized and measured in identical ways across studies" (Redeker et al., 2015, p. 379), but CDEs reach further into clinical practice. Patient-Reported Outcomes Measurement Information System (PROMIS; Northwestern University, 2018) is a person-centric outcome measure that has clear definitions and methods of documentation. One example is categorization of pain. PROMIS has a three-question method to determine the intensity and level of pain. PROMIS is only one method of standardized patient outcome measures. The Agency for Healthcare Research and Quality (AHRQ), a component of the federal government, supports research to improve healthcare quality. The AHRQ recommends standardizing outcome measures to ensure increased quality and decreased healthcare costs through the use of the National Quality Measures Clearinghouse (NQMC) database housing standardized healthcare quality measures (Box 8.3). The AHRQ NQMC's mission is to provide evidence of healthcare safety, quality, accessibility, equitability, and affordability (Agency for Healthcare Research and Quality [AHRQ], 2014). They also support the implementation and dissemination of healthcare information as an adjunct to increasing and improving patient/provider decision-making.

Patient care is a multidisciplinary task. Beyond nursing, interdisciplinary teams function better and patient outcomes are improved when documentation is standardized across disciplines. Consider the example of the Kaiser Permanente Delirium Initiative. Exploring the clinical problem of delirium led to knowledge that nursing-generated delirium assessment data were not visible to physicians writing medication orders; pharmacists aware of the deliriogenic properties of medications were unable to see that patients were at risk for or experiencing delirium (Soriano, Chow, & O'Brien, 2017).

BOX 8.3

AHRQ HEALTH QUALITY INDICATORS

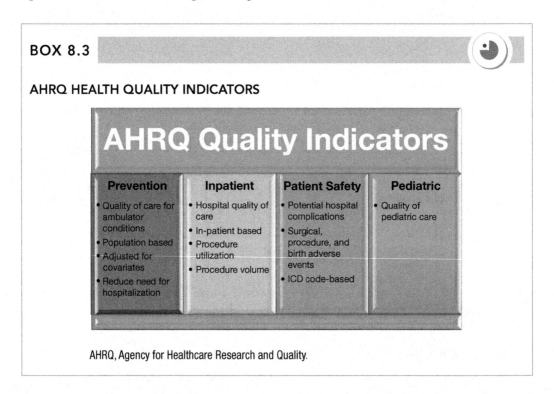

AHRQ, Agency for Healthcare Research and Quality.

After identifying these systems shortfalls, the interdisciplinary team developed a machine-readable risk score based on patient characteristics, nursing assessment data, medications, surgical status, and other elements already present in the EHR. This interdisciplinary score increased transparency between providers and provided decision-making support at the point of care for nurses, physicians, and pharmacists to reduce the risk for and consequences of delirium. By standardizing the data entered by each clinical discipline and integrating that data into real-time knowledge, initiatives like the Kaiser Permanente Delirium Initiative have the potential to greatly improve both patient outcomes and nursing workflow.

Questions to Consider Before Reading On

1. *How can nursing data be standardized across providers? Units? Healthcare systems?*

2. *What are two of the functions that standardized data support?*

Documentation Requirements

The American Nurses Association (ANA, 2010) describes documentation as an essential component of high-quality, evidence-based nursing care. Documentation is often derided as cumbersome, time-consuming, and in competition with direct patient care. Yet maintaining accurate, timely, and accessible patient records serves a number of vital functions that lead to improved outcomes for patients within and across systems:

- Improves communication between nurses and across disciplines
- Facilitates communication and comparison across healthcare settings and systems
- Enables auditing for purposes of accreditation, credentialing, and legal inquiry
- Supports legislation and regulatory compliance
- Improves accuracy of reimbursement and cost analysis
- Provides valuable clinical data for research and quality improvement

The ANA (2010) describes six principles of high-quality nursing documentation (Box 8.4). The sixth principle of high-quality nursing documentation, Standardized Terminologies, requires professional nurses to be familiar with sources of standardized language specific to nursing and accepted for use across healthcare systems and organizations.

BOX 8.4

ESSENTIAL PRINCIPLES OF NURSING DOCUMENTATION

Principle 1: Documentation characteristics	High-quality documentation is: accurate, timely, relevant, consistent, accessible, auditable, permanent, clear, concise, complete, legible, thoughtful, and reflective of the nursing process
Principle 2: Education and training	Nurses should be trained and competent at technical aspects of documentation (e.g., documentation software, computers)
Principle 3: Policies and procedures	Nurses should be trained and familiar with institutional policies and procedures related to documentation

(continued)

BOX 8.4 (*continued*)

Principle 4: Protection systems	Systems must be in place to protect data and provide confidentiality of patient, provider, and institutional information
Principle 5: Documentation entries	Entries must be timely, legible, authenticated, accurate, complete, date and time stamped by the person making the entry
Principle 6: Standardized terminologies	High-quality documentation uses standardized terminologies, including acronyms and symbols, so that data may be aggregated across settings

These standards are put into place to provide transparency of patient-related information. Early in the development and adoption of EHR systems, the Department of Health and Human Services (DHHS) Office of the National Coordinator for Health Information Technology (ONC, 2018) required that to receive financial assistance for the expensive task of putting EHRs into use, patient-related data must be used meaningfully, in other words shared. Meaningful use also required that EHRs adopt Systemized Nomenclature of Medicine (SNOMED), a multilingual standardized terminology bank, to assure standardization of clinical terminology (Box 8.5).

BOX 8.5

DATA STANDARDIZATION: SOURCES OF STANDARDIZED LANGUAGE IN NURSING DOCUMENTATION

STANDARDIZATION SOURCES	
Logical Observation Identifiers Names and Codes (LOINC)[a]	LOINC, created and maintained by the Regenstrief Institute, is a universal database identifying medical laboratory observations.
Nursing Minimum Data Set (NMDS)[b]	The NMDS is a classification system, now incorporated into LOINC, that provides a standardized collection of essential nursing data.
Systematized Nomenclature of Medicine-CT—Clinical Terms (SNOMED-CT)[c]	SNOMED-CT is a standardized, multilingual vocabulary of clinical terminology used by healthcare providers to electronically share/exchange clinical health information.

(continued)

BOX 8.5 (*continued*)

STANDARDIZATION SOURCES	
Nursing Interventions Classification (NIC) and the Nursing Outcomes Classification (NOC)[d]	NIC NOC is an ANA-approved standardized classification system of nursing-sensitive patient outcomes. These classifications provide terminology describing nursing judgments, treatments, and nursing-sensitive patient outcomes.

[a]https://loinc.org

[b]Werley, H. H., Devine, E. C., Zorn, C. R., Ryan, P., & Westra, B. L. (1991). The nursing minimum data set: Abstraction tool for standardized, comparable, essential data. *American Journal of Public Health, 81*(4), 421–426. doi:10.2105/ajph.81.4.421

[c]https://www.snomed.org/snomed-ct

[d]http://www.nanda.org/nanda-i-nic-noc.html

ANA, American Nurses Association.

Standardization allows EHR data to be used for continuous quality improvement and research, yet room remains for customization of EHR systems to account for diverse patient populations and workflows. In many cases, the adoption of standardized language and machine-readable documentation enables customized fields and workflows to be combined in a meaningful way despite differences in how data are presented within EHRs. For example, physicians might be provided with a view that automatically displays standardized nursing documentation related to blood glucose monitoring and insulin administration when writing orders for dietary changes in diabetic patients. Nurses may have a screen to automatically notify pharmacy and physicians when adverse reactions are documented against medications.

Data harmonization, or the process of integrating diverse data into a single system, allows similar data that are coded differently across systems to be combined for aggregate uses (Bowles et al., 2013). For example, pain assessment data using a visual scale in hospital A might be harmonized with a 1 to 10 verbal rating scale used in hospital B so that comparisons across settings can be made. This allows researchers and quality improvement teams to sample patients from multiple settings to obtain more generalizable and accurate information on health, particularly in patients who have rare conditions or specialized needs.

Such aggregation is the foundation for precision health initiatives, allowing researchers to identify risk and protective factors that influence outcomes in diverse groups of patients. The Common Data Model (Box 8.6) shows how data harmonization occurs when documentation needs vary across settings.

BOX 8.6

OBSERVATIONAL MEDICAL OUTCOMES PARTNERSHIP COMMON DATA MODEL—A GRAPHICAL REPRESENTATION OF THE PROCESS OF STANDARDIZING DATA ACROSS DIVERSE SETTINGS FOR RESEARCH

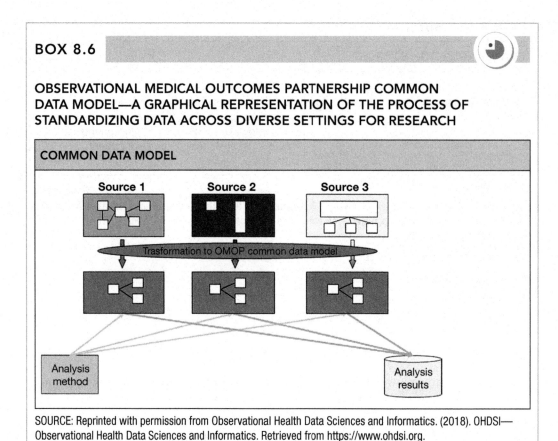

SOURCE: Reprinted with permission from Observational Health Data Sciences and Informatics. (2018). OHDSI—Observational Health Data Sciences and Informatics. Retrieved from https://www.ohdsi.org.

Let us consider again the example of harmonizing pain scales discussed earlier. If each "source" in the model is a hospital system and the boxes within each source represent common types of patient data (e.g., pain assessments, medication administration records, diagnoses), then to harmonize the data, it would first have to be converted to a single structure. In this case that conversion is presented by the common data model. The common data model provides a structure for organizing data from diverse sources into a single format. Once the data are in the same format, computers and researchers can quickly access and analyze trends, patterns, and relationships between and within systems, producing analysis results that are comparable.

■ Question to Consider Before Reading On

1. *In what way does using nursing informatics improve patient outcomes?*

Nursing Informatics in Practice

Nurses in the clinical setting can improve the usefulness of nursing and patient data from EHR systems by advocating for the adoption and use of standardized terminology and machine-readable nursing documentation. Professional nurses are empowered by nursing informatics knowledge about data standardization to advocate for and assist in the development and maintenance of standardized data collection, curation, and management. By using nursing's strong documentation and patient characterization skills in a standardized, machine-readable way that is accessible beyond the bedside, nurses have the potential to improve patient outcomes across healthcare settings and systems (Porter, Larsson, & Lee, 2016).

Questions to Consider Before Reading On

1. *What documentation standards are used in your facility?*
2. *How do documentation standards improve patient safety?*

Outcomes of Data Standardization

For the individual patient, data standardization and the use of machine-readable documentation allow closer monitoring of changes over time and graphical representation of patient trends (Box 8.7).

BOX 8.7

GRAPHICAL REPRESENTATION OF PATIENT DATA TRENDS

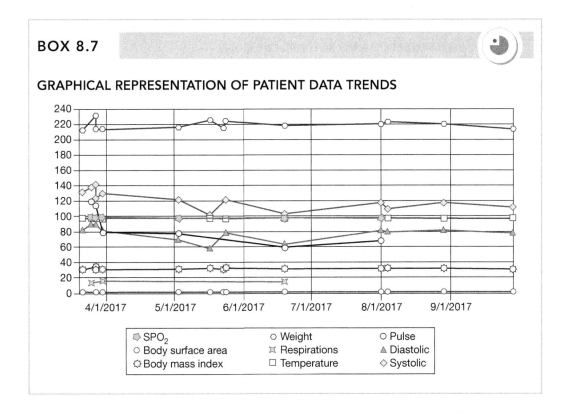

Legend:
- ⇨ SPO$_2$
- ○ Body surface area
- ✿ Body mass index
- ○ Weight
- ⋈ Respirations
- ☐ Temperature
- ○ Pulse
- ▲ Diastolic
- ◇ Systolic

Close monitoring of patient trends is a critical step in the prevention of failure to rescue, which occurs when providers miss or fail to prevent complications of medical care and which often result in cardiorespiratory failure and unnecessary death (AHRQ, 2017).

For healthcare providers and organizations, improved documentation insures appropriate reimbursement, easing financial strains that can lead to understaffing and inadequate reinvestment. Standardization and improved access to patient information for diverse healthcare providers have direct implications for patient safety, preventing medication errors associated with polypharmacy and reducing financial burdens on patients from repeated testing. They also improve healthcare quality by insuring that diverse providers are aware of one another's findings and treatments and providing decision support for clinical decision-making.

Beyond the bedside, standardization also reduces time and workload on support staff and managers required to compile accreditation and legal documentation in compliance with professional standards and legislative requirements, freeing up time for more staff- and patient-centered activities. This enables improvements in healthcare settings, systems, and disciplinary standards of care. The primary goal of the DHHS directive on meaningful use of EHR data is to allow continuous quality improvement and research to improve patient outcomes (ONC, 2018; Porter, Larsson, & Lee, 2016). This goal is compatible with the goal of nursing to provide high-quality care through evidence-based practice.

QSEN SCENARIO

The goals of nursing are to increase patient quality, reduce error, and protect patient safety. Standardization of documentation and information is one method to support these goals by improving patient safety and healthcare quality.

How would you be a champion for technologies that support clinical decision making that meet the aforementioned goals while protecting patient privacy?

■ Question to Consider Before Reading On

1. *What is the role of quality improvement in clinical practice?*
2. *What is an advantage of applying standardized data to clinical practice?*

Research conducted through EHR records provides critical evidence upon which to build policies, procedures, and practice change initiatives. Quality improvement initiatives provide ongoing evidence of the efficacy and impact of evidence-based practice change on real-world settings and allow continuous adjustment to enhance patient safety and well-being. The availability of standardized data and CDEs reduces the cost and time-consumption of research and quality improvement projects (Redeker et al., 2015), leading to a more rapid expansion of nursing knowledge and improved quality for patients.

Critical Thinking Questions and Activities

Take a few minutes to review your practice setting's documentation policies.

- *What type of standardization goals are in place?*
- *How might these be improved to enhance the usefulness of nursing-generated data?*

Discuss documentation with a colleague working in another discipline.

- *Are nursing documentation and data easy to find and view by physicians, respiratory therapists, and other members of the healthcare team?*
- *Can nurses access, locate, and easily review documentation by other disciplines?*

SUMMARY

In conclusion, data standardization supports the goals of nursing to improve direct patient care and healthcare safety and quality. By allowing comparison of patients across healthcare systems and settings, data standardization has the potential to enhance the evidence basis for nursing practice and to improve clinical outcomes. Data standardization has the potential to decrease the costs of healthcare to patients and organizations by improving reimbursement, decreasing unnecessary testing, and streamlining the processes like nursing and physician documentation, giving providers more time to care for patients directly. Professional nurses with knowledge of data standardization are empowered to advocate on behalf of the discipline and patients to improve machine readability of nursing documentation and to improve care.

References

Agency for Healthcare Research and Quality. (2014). Mission and budget. Retrieved from https://www.ahrq.gov/cpi/about/mission/index.html

Agency for Healthcare Research and Quality. (2017). Failure to rescue. Retrieved from https://psnet.ahrq.gov/primers/primer/38/failure-to-rescue

American Nurses Association. (2010). *ANA's principles for nursing documentation: Guidance for registered nurses.* Silver Spring, MD: Author. Retrieved from https://www.nursingworld.org/globalassets/docs/ana/ethics/principles-of-nursing-documentation.pdf

Bowles, K., Potashnik, S., Ratcliffe, S., Rosenberg, M., Shih, N.-W., Topaz, M., ... Naylor, M. (2013). Conducting research using the electronic health record across multi-hospital systems: Semantic harmonization implications for administrators. *The Journal of Nursing Administration, 43*(6), 355–360. doi:10.1097/nna.0b013e3182942c3c

IBM (2015). Standardized data: Definition - IBM. Retrieved from https://www.ibm.com/support/knowledgecenter/en/SSWSR9_11.6.0/com.ibm.mdshs.initiateglossary.doc/topics/r_glossary_standardized_data.html

Northwestern University. (2018). PROMIS. Retrieved from http://www.healthmeasures.net/explore-measurement-systems/promis

Observational Health Data Sciences and Informatics. (2018). OHDSI—Observational Health Data Sciences and Informatics. Retrieved from https://www.ohdsi.org

Office of the National Coordinator for Health Information Technology. (2018). Meaningful use and MACRA. Retrieved from https://www.healthit.gov/topic/meaningful-use-and -macra/meaningful-use-and-macra

Porter, M. E., Larsson, S., & Lee, T. H. (2016). Standardizing patient outcome measurement. *New England Journal of Medicine, 374,* 504–506. doi:10.1056/NEJMp1511701

Redeker, N. S., Anderson, R., Bakken, S., Corwin, E., Docherty, S., Dorsey, S. G., … Grady, P. (2015). Advancing symptom science through use of common data elements. *Journal of Nursing Scholarship, 47*(5), 379–388. doi:10.1111/jnu.12155

Soriano, R., Chow, M., & O'Brien, A. (2017). Leveraging the power of interprofessional EHR data to prevent delirium: The Kaiser Permanente story. In *Big data-enabled nursing education, research and practice* (pp. 301–312). Cham, Switzerland: Springer International.

CHAPTER 9

NURSING INFORMATICS: BIG DATA APPLICATIONS TO INFORM PRACTICE

LYNDA HARDY | LISA M. BLAIR

LEARNING OBJECTIVES AND OUTCOMES

Upon completion of this chapter, the reader will be able to:

- Define big data.
- Define data science.
- Identify the DIKW model and its application to nursing.
- Identify two outcomes for how data informs practice.

⊙ KEY NURSING INFORMATICS TERMS

Some of the key concepts and terms you will hear in this chapter are:

Analytics

Big data

Big Data to Knowledge (BD2K)

Data

Data science

Data, Information, Knowledge, Wisdom (DIKW) model

Healthcare Information and Management Systems Society (HIMSS)

Information

Knowledge

Technology Informatics Guiding Education Reform (TIGER)

Variety

Velocity

Veracity

Volume

Wisdom

INTRODUCTION

Florence Nightingale knew about the power of data as she cared for soldiers in the Crimean War. She understood the need to document what she was doing to determine how components of her work affected the patients she cared for. Nightingale described and analyzed variables such as ventilation, warmth, noise, food, light, and cleanliness and their effect on patient outcomes. She knew that documentation and analysis were key to patient care, quality, and safety (Nightingale, 1969).

Since Nightingale's direction, nursing continues to grow as a discipline, increasing fundamental and expert practices. As defined by the International Council of Nurses (2018), nursing "encompasses autonomous and collaborative care of individuals of all ages, families, groups and communities, sick or well, and in all settings. Nursing includes the promotion of health, prevention of illness, and the care of ill, disabled, and dying people. Advocacy, promotion of a safe environment, research, participation in shaping health policy and in patient and health systems management, and education are also key nursing roles." The performance of nursing requires a complete understanding of patient healthcare needs resulting from interdisciplinary data and information collected by an ongoing process.

Today, as a practicing nurse you understand the need to "document" patient care, but the importance of that documentation lies in the understanding that the *data* can be collected across time to provide *information* that provides *knowledge* to the healthcare team, leading to *wisdom* regarding how to care for the patient. *Data, information, knowledge, wisdom (DIKW)!*

▓ Questions to Consider Before Reading On

1. *What is the DIKW model? How can it be applied to clinical practice?*
2. *What is the difference between data and datum?*
3. *What healthcare "data" do you currently collect?*
4. *What do you or your patients wear that helps collect data to help inform health and healthcare?*
5. *What other data and information do you use for patient care?*

▓ What Is the Data-Information-Knowledge-Wisdom (DIKW) Model?

There are many uses and descriptions of the interdisciplinary DIKW model discussed in previous chapters (Figure 9.1). The DIKW model depicts four independent steps of a process that turns data into actionable wisdom and practice change.

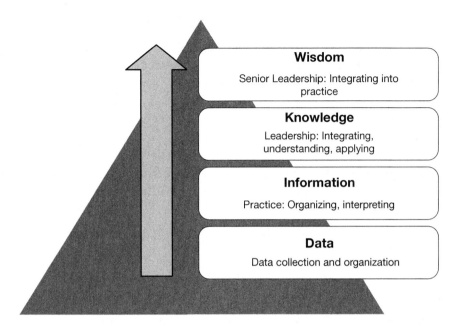

FIGURE 9.1 Data, information, knowledge, and wisdom (DIKW) hierarchy for nursing.

SOURCE: Adapted from Staggers, N., & Nelson, R. (2015). Data, information, knowledge, wisdom. In S. J. Henly (Ed.), *Routledge international handbook of advanced quantitative methods in nursing research*. New York, NY: Routledge.

Defining Data

It all starts with data. First, the word "data" is plural; a singular piece of data is a "datum." A datum is the beginning point in healthcare. Each datum provides little information, but taken together, data provide points that can be used in aggregation to answer questions or provide trends for patient outcomes.

Healthcare data can be defined as facts collected on patients and services used across the entire healthcare system. The continual creation of healthcare data makes it difficult to determine the amount of data generated every day.

One IBM report suggests that 2.5 quintillion units of electronic data are generated daily (IBM, 2017)—that is a lot of data! The DIKW hierarchy shows that collecting and organizing data into a usable form results in the creation of information.

Datum Examples: A single point
- Patient temperature
- Diastolic blood pressure measurement
- Respiratory measurement

Defining Information

Data are aggregated and processed in the information stage of the DIKW model. Data relationships become more evident as the pieces of the patient care puzzle continue to be put into place. Nursing professionals collect large amounts of data daily on patients, service, and staffing that are transformed into information through organizing and interpreting the data. The information highlights patient data trends and health system factors that could influence patient care or practice.

Defining Knowledge

Knowledge is the third level of the DIKW model. This step continues the process of understanding the information that has been gathered to allow nursing leadership to further interpret the information and apply it more broadly. Knowledge is when data and information are used to identify relationships.

Defining Wisdom

The last step in the DIKW hierarchy is wisdom. Knowledge, in this step, is applied and integrated into the workflow and patient care system. Wisdom provides leaders the "why" of the information and knowledge and indicates the need and type of more global steps to be undertaken. This culminates the DIKW model to show how data can be converted into actionable results based on wisdom.

Linking the DIKW to Nursing Process

The DIKW model has similarities to the nursing process (Figure 9.2). Nurses obtain data about their patients that provide information leading to knowledge of patient needs to inform care. Wisdom is an abstract concept that is the culmination of knowledge.

The acquisition of data requires assessment of the patient, health system, and/or care environment. Organizing and aggregating the data into information allow us to identify trends and diagnose problems. Further processing information to create knowledge is similar to the planning phase of the nursing process, in that we are planning how to act in response to our diagnosed problems. Finally, we implement practice or systems changes that address the problems by acting on the wisdom we gain from the data. The DIKW model, like the nursing process, is iterative in nature, meaning that once we implement the changes suggested by our newfound wisdom, we continue to seek new DIKW to support our changes or to suggest new directions for improvement in patient care, safety, workflow, productivity, and health systems.

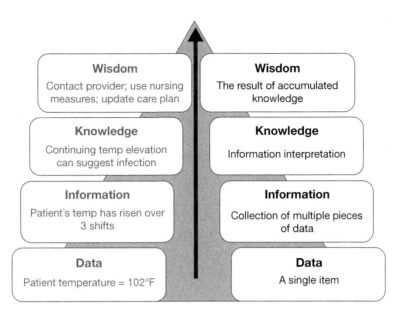

FIGURE 9.2 Nursing and DIKW—Applying the DIKW model to nursing practice—an exemplar.

DIKW, data, information, knowledge, wisdom.

Questions to Consider Before Reading On

1. *What is big data?*
2. *What are the five characteristics of data?*
3. *What is data science? Why is it important to understand and apply these concepts?*

Defining Big Data and Data Science

The term "big data" was originally coined by researchers seeking to describe the difficulties of working with the vast arrays of data generated by fluid dynamics tests (Cox & Ellsworth, 1997). Recently, the healthcare industry experienced a data explosion that continues to grow. The development and expansion of electronic health records plus the proliferation of equipment capable of collecting real-time patient data in a structured form have increased the pace and size of incoming data about patients, nursing, healthcare organizations, and the healthcare system.

The five major characteristics described in Figure 9.3 suggest that big data must be looked at in terms of its relationship to the need. Big data is a challenge with enormous potential to improve patient outcomes and nursing workflows, but we, as healthcare providers, must understand its volume, variety, velocity, veracity, and value (IBM, 2014). Each of these characteristics requires specialized expertise, equipment, and analytic procedures.

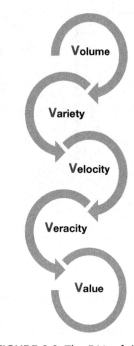

FIGURE 9.3 The 5 Vs of data.

- **Volume** describes the scale of data that requires advanced computing capacity to store and process.
- **Variety** highlights the wide range of data types that are input, from narrative notes to cardiopulmonary monitor data to imaging.
- **Velocity** in the healthcare context describes the fast pace of incoming data from individual patients, clinicians, and healthcare facilities and systems across the country and around the world.
- **Veracity**, or trustworthiness of the information, relates to measurement error, missing data points, and other sources of uncertainty inherent in such large-scale data that require special handling. In healthcare literature, value, or the usefulness of the data, is often added to this list of big data characteristics (Brennan & Bakken, 2015).
- **Value** relates to what the data mean to us. Enormous amounts of data can be collected but we must assure that the data we do collect are meaningful.

Data science is an emerging scientific field dedicated to working with data on all scales and of many types and employing expertise curated from a wide range of traditional scientific fields for the purpose of improving decision making, accelerating innovation, and enhancing access to data-driven knowledge (Brennan & Bakken, 2015). Data scientists come from a variety of backgrounds and fields and have multiple pathways to the expertise that allows them to effectively organize, analyze, and interpret data or turn data into knowledge.

Just like other industries struggling to deal with the flood of incoming data (Snibbe, 2006), nursing is at risk of "drowning in data" (p. 39) without appropriate data science expertise. Nurse leaders, including the director of the National Library of Medicine, Patricia Brennan, have called for nurses to embrace big data and data science, from the bedside to the national policy stage (Brennan & Bakken, 2015).

Similarly, the National Institutes of Health's Big Data to Knowledge (BD2K) initiative invested over $200 million to improve the access of nursing to the benefits of big data and data science through research and the funding and support of data sciences (National Institutes of Health, 2018).

Data continue to grow at unimaginable rates. Healthcare data grow exponentially as health information technology, such as electronic health records and wearable devices, grows. We are increasing our ability to use various types of healthcare analytical methods, such as healthcare research, the patient experience, continuing care, prevention and prediction to better inform patient care and outcomes (Stanford University, 2017).

Big data and data science offer the potential for big value to patients, healthcare systems, and society, but with big value comes added risk of breaches of confidentiality and patient privacy. Hacking, data breaches, and cybersecurity lapses pose serious ethical concerns and technological challenges that will continue to adapt and advance in the coming years.

We, as nurses who collect, curate, and interpret data, are charged with the added burden of protecting patient confidentiality and privacy in settings where data are ubiquitous.

Nurses engaged in quality improvement and research may have access to vast volumes of patient data, requiring special security to adequately protect. Issues around informed consent, privacy, and anonymity have been raised in conjunction with big data science practices in nursing (Milton, 2017).

Ethicists will likely continue to wrestle with balancing the potential value to society against individual rights to privacy and autonomy in the context of big data and data analysis. Nurses must play a key role in the development of ethical guidelines around the use of patient data if our disciplinary perspective on the patient-centeredness of care is to be acknowledged and maintained.

▓ Questions to Consider Before Reading On

1. *What is HIMSS's definition of nursing informatics?*
2. *What is one example of how use of data and nursing informatics leads to improved patient care?*

DIKW, Data Science, and Nursing Informatics

Considering the previous information, one could say that all nurses are data scientists and informaticists. Nurses, on a daily basis, review patient information through dashboards on electronic health records. They determine patient trends in anticipation of describing patient needs through nursing diagnoses and interventions. They consult the patient's data to assist in decision making both with the patient and with nursing colleagues. Nurses rely on data and information to provide the appropriate knowledge that will increase the quality of the care they provide and decrease potential patient-related errors.

Nursing informatics is a specialty area that delves deeper into data. Healthcare Information and Management Systems Society (HIMSS) defines nursing informatics as "the specialty that integrates nursing science with multiple information management and analytical sciences to identify, define, manage, and communicate data, information, knowledge, and wisdom in nursing practice" (HIMSS, 2015; www.himss.org/what-nursing-informatics). The American Nursing Informatics Association provides guidance and insight into the depth and breadth of nursing informatics, suggesting that nurse informaticists work to develop and communicate information technologies. They act as educators, researchers, and nursing and community leaders who use health informatics to advance healthcare.

CASE SCENARIO

DATA USE IN NURSING

An 8-year-old child is admitted to the emergency room (ER) with difficulty breathing. The ER nurse is able to search hospital records, locating a previous ER visit for this child. She reviewed the information noting that tests were performed for allergy determination and noted that the child was allergic to tree pollen.

1. What questions might the ER nurse ask the mother regarding any previous visits or episodes with difficulty breathing to begin her medical records search?

The nurse further checked geographical data on tree pollen levels that day and found them to be at extremely high levels.

2. Where would the nurse search to retrieve current, relevant data for pollen levels?

The electronic medical record (EHR) further noted that the child was successfully treated with nebulizer treatments followed up by a steroid-based inhaler. She notified the attending physician about her findings and the child was treated rapidly for targeted care.

3. Where would the nurse search in the EHR to determine previous treatments that were successful?

■ Questions to Consider Before Reading On

1. *What is one example of how use of data and integrating it into practice using nursing informatics skills can improve clinical practice?*

2. *How is precision medicine applied?*

Outcomes of Integrating Big Data, Data Science, and DIKW Into Practice

Exemplar 1

A classic example of the application of the DIKW model can be found in NICU nursing (Brown, 2009). The NICU patient data were collected about hearing loss via newborn hearing screening and auditory testing. At the same time, data were collected about environmental noise from monitors, ventilators, alarms, speaking voices, and other sources in the NICU environment.

These data were organized and aggregated to produce two important pieces of information:

1. NICU patients had high rates of hearing loss, and
2. NICU environments had noise well above thresholds for hearing damage.

By examining the relationship between hearing loss and noise levels, researchers discovered that there was a strong correlation between noisy NICU environments and permanent hearing damage in patients. This knowledge was then translated into wisdom through practice changes (e.g., silencing monitors, reducing alarm volumes, insulating sound equipment) and environmental changes (e.g., placing noise sensors on units that light up when excessive noise is present to alert staff, covering isolettes with blankets to insulate infants from noise).

Big data has, on a larger scale, been integrated into practice for decades in the form of large-scale epidemiological studies that have identified sources of infectious disease and environmental risk. Information on disease prevalence and incidence is curated and analyzed by national organizations such as the Centers for Disease Control and Prevention (CDC) to inform clinicians and monitor public health and safety. Research findings from large national surveys such as the National Health and Nutrition Examination Survey (CDC, 2018) have highlighted health risks and protective factors for conditions as disparate as obesity and lead toxicity.

These trends in the use of big data to improve human health are increasing in pace and complexity. For example, the National Institutes of Health (2018) launched a precision medicine initiative to measure and monitor the genetic, biological, psychological, environmental, and general health measures of 1 million people! This health initiative seeks to build knowledge and wisdom to affect the health of people across the United States and across the globe.

QSEN SCENARIO

QSEN informatics competencies require that nurses have the ability to "Identify essential information that must be available in a common database to support patient care." EHR provides patient data and information for providers.

1. What elements of the EHR would you use to determine patient data and information?
2. How would you use the information to support patient care?
3. How do data help nurses and patients make clinical decisions?

CASE SCENARIO (CONTINUED)

The 8-year-old child admitted to the emergency room with difficulty breathing noted to be an allergic response to environmental allergies responded well to the nebulizer treatments. The nurse caring for the child further reviewed the child's EHR, noting previous parent and child asthma education. She discussed that education with the patient and the parent to determine effectiveness, noting that the child was interested more in technology than in paper teaching.

The nurse is aware of health information technology games (education gamification) that assist children and adolescents in staying involved in their care while using mHealth-related games. She introduces a reliable and valid asthma-related mobile application to the parent and child as a method of increasing the child's needs for asthma self-care. The application will alert the child when asthma triggers are high and provide methods for the child to reduce their impact. The questions and considerations the nurse explored to gain this information were as follows:

1. What type of data do you collect either in practice or personally?
2. How do these data affect how you care for patients or yourself?
3. How would you consider using data and information going forward?
4. What concerns do you have about the use of individual patient data in large data sets?

◾ Questions to Consider Before Reading On

1. *What do nurses need to know about data to better patient care?*
2. *What educational skills and competencies are required of nurses?*

◾ Critical Thinking Questions and Activities

QUESTION	ACTIVITY
What type of patient information is included in your facility's EHR?	Review your facility's EHR carefully looking at your patient's dashboard to determine what information exists to help in determining patient care.
What health information technology support systems exist in your facility's EHR?	If you are uncertain about the response to this question, ask your unit supervisor what systems are included in the EHR and how to access them. Inquire if the system is a Clinical Decision System that assists in patient care.
What methods do you use to protect patient healthcare information?	Having the ability to see patient information is not only essential for patient care but also important to understand how to protect the patient's data. If you are not familiar with health information policies at your facility, contact your supervisor or the chief information officer to assure that, during patient care, you are fully protecting your patients.

▨ Critical Thinking Questions and Competency Activities

President George W. Bush outlined a plan, in 2004, that by 2014 every American would have EHR. This set in motion a series of events that supported the need for education related to informatics. Healthcare providers, information technologists, hospitals, and payers form the Technology Informatics Guiding Education Reform (TIGER) team to consider the amount and level of information technology education required for providers (Shaw, Sensmeier, & Anderson, 2017). The TIGER team worked through three phases and iterations of the necessary education to better inform healthcare providers about health information technology. Today, a list of TIGER competencies can be found through the HIMSS at www.tigercompetencies.pbworks.com/w/page/22247287/FrontPage.

■ *What are three of the basic computer competencies suggested in this article?*

Nursing leaders continue to review educational requirements for health information, suggesting that education should include a number of basic computer skills, such as software, electronic communication, data access, patient-related application, and informatics knowledge, such as management concepts, data issues, information concepts, clinical research, and ethical and legal issues (Westra & Delaney, 2008). The American Association of Colleges of Nursing (2008) inserted informatics competencies into *The Essentials of Baccalaureate Education for Professional Nursing*.

■ *The QSEN Institute (2018) noted informatics as one of its six core competencies. Conduct a search of the QSEN website: www.qsen.org/competencies/pre-licensure -ksas. <Scroll down> Find the Informatics section; List two skills/competencies expected of a prelicensure nurse.*

SUMMARY

Bringing it All Together!

The magnitude and pace of data often make it overwhelming. There is a need to understand new terminologies, to learn new and ever-changing devices, and to protect the patient information that we, as nurses, have access to.

Nursing practice and the infusion of informatics and data science into that practice provide challenges for new and experienced nurses. Data, information, and knowledge provide the wisdom to assist healthcare professionals make clinical decisions about patient care. The DIKW model provides patient insight from the 10,000 foot level down to the 10 foot level, providing healthcare providers a deep dive into the patient's health, the course it has been on, and a possible map going forward. The importance of patient information increases the need to safeguard that data, posing additional challenges in the context of the high value of individual patient data when aggregated. We as nurses have an ethical code to provide a framework for patient care and protection and to guard the health, safety, and rights of patients and governance of their information.

If we keep in mind the DIKW model with the understanding of responsibility at each level, nursing will continue to embrace the power of data as a means of bettering patient outcomes with tools that increase patient safety, patient care quality, and patient satisfaction.

■ References

American Association of Colleges of Nursing. (2008). The essentials of baccalaureate education for professional nursing practice. Retrieved from https://www.aacnnursing.org/Education-Resources/AACN-Essentials

Brennan, P. F., & Bakken, S. (2015). Nursing needs big data and big data needs nursing. *Journal of Nursing Scholarship*, *47*(5), 477–484. doi:10.1111/jnu.12159

Brown, G. (2009). NICU noise and the preterm infant. *Neonatal Network: NN*, *28*(3), 165–173. doi:10.1891/0730-0832.28.3.165

Centers for Disease Control and Prevention. (2018). NHANES—National Health and Nutrition Examination Survey homepage. Retrieved from https://www.cdc.gov/nchs/nhanes/index.htm

Cox, M., & Ellsworth, D. (1997). Application-controlled demand paging for out-of-core visualization. *Proceedings of the 8th Conference on Visualization '97*, Phoenix, AZ, 235–244. doi:10.1145/266989.267068

Healthcare Information and Management Systems Society. (2015). Nursing informatics. Retrieved from http://www.himss.org/what-nursing-informatics

International Business Machines. (2014). The four V's of big data. Retrieved from http://www.ibmbigdatahub.com/infographic/four-vs-big-data

International Business Machines (2017). *2017 annual report*. https://www.ibm.com/annualreport/2017/assets/downloads/IBM_Annual_Report_2017.pdf

International Council of Nurses. (2018). Definition of nursing. Retrieved from http://www.icn.ch/who-we-are/icn-definition-of-nursing

Milton, C. L. (2017). The ethics of big data and nursing science. *Nursing Science Quarterly*, *30*(4), 300–302. doi:10.1177/0894318417724474

National Institutes of Health. (2018). Big data to knowledge. *NIH Common Fund*. Retrieved from https://commonfund.nih.gov/bd2k

Nightingale, F. (1969). *Notes on nursing: What it is, and what it is not*. New York, NY: Dover.

QSEN Institute. (2018). Competencies. Retrieved from http://qsen.org/competencies

Shaw, T., Sensmeier, J., & Anderson, C. (2017). The evolution of the TIGER initiative. *CIN: Computers, Informatics, Nursing*, *35*(6), 278–280. doi:10.1097/CIN.0000000000000369

Snibbe, A. C. (2006). Drowning in data. *Stanford Social Innovation Review*, 39–45.

Staggers, N., & Nelson, R. (2015). Data, information, knowledge, wisdom. In S. J. Henly (Ed.), *Routledge international handbook of advanced quantitative methods in nursing research*. New York, NY: Routledge.

Stanford University. (2017). *Harnessing the power of data in health*. Retrieved from https://med.stanford.edu/content/dam/sm/sm-news/documents/StanfordMedicineHealthTrendsWhitePaper2017.pdf

Westra, B. L., & Delaney, C. W. (2008). Informatics competencies for nursing and healthcare leaders (pp. 804–808). In *AMIA Annual Symposium Proceedings. Westra BL1, Delaney CW*: American Medical Informatics Association.

PART V

NURSING INFORMATICS: MANAGING QUALITY, ASSESSMENT, AND EVALUATION

CHAPTER 10

NURSING INFORMATICS: MAINTAINING QUALITY OF DATA AND INFORMATION

TONI HEBDA | KATHLEEN HUNTER

LEARNING OBJECTIVES AND OUTCOMES

Upon completion of this chapter, the reader will be able to:

- Identify the attributes required for quality data and information.
- Explain ways in which the nurse can ensure the quality of data and information.
- Describe the significance of the quality of data and information for clinical practice, patient outcomes, and the body of nursing knowledge.
- Discuss the relationships between information management and the quality of data and information.
- Discuss the relationship between quality of data and information and outcomes expected of graduates of nursing programs as identified by the American Association of Colleges of Nursing.
- Explain the relationship between quality of data and information and competencies expected of the professional nurse as identified by the Quality and Safety Education for Nurses (QSEN) project.
- Identify informatics competencies expected of professional nurses that relate to the quality of data and information.

⊙ KEY NURSING INFORMATICS TERMS

Data integrity

Data quality

Data scrubbing or cleansing

Data silo

Data validation

Information management

Information quality

INTRODUCTION

Chapter 2 discussed the data-information-knowledge-wisdom (DIKW) framework, providing definitions for the individual concepts of data, information, knowledge, and wisdom as well as examples of how one applies those same concepts each day. The DIKW framework works well when one begins with a solid foundation of quality data that are available when and where they are needed by the persons who need it. That, however, is the ideal situation, and not every situation is ideal.

This chapter focuses on maintaining the quality of data and information, starting with what determines quality, actions that the individual nurse can take to ensure quality, computer applications of data and information in practice, and expectations defined by the AACN in the *Essentials* documents for graduates of nursing programs and the QSEN project for the professional nurse as they relate to data and information use and management in practice.

■ Questions to Consider Before Reading On

1. *List three attributes of quality data.*
2. *What does* accurate *mean?*

■ What Is Quality Data?

In very general terms, quality data meet requirements that have been predetermined. However, the broad nature of this definition makes it difficult to say exactly what quality data is. Complete, correct, and accurate are commonly identified attributes of good data. *Complete* means you have all the values or characteristics together. *Correct* means the data or information is a true, valid indicator of an entity or phenomenon. For example, a systolic blood pressure reading would give a number without decimal values. *Accurate* refers to the value being the actual measured value. For example, if a person's name is Albert Einstein, the name is always shown as Albert Einstein.

In healthcare, it is also critical that data be available on demand (when), at the right location (where), and to the persons who need it (who; Stausberg, Nasseh, & Nonnemacher, 2015). For a discussion of more quality attributes, see the article by Strausber et al.

■ Questions to Consider Before Reading On

1. *What does* garbage in, garbage out, *mean with regard to quality information?*
2. *Discuss five attributes of quality data.*

■ What Is Quality Information?

Information is built on data, so information quality (IQ) is dependent on data quality. It is highly unlikely that quality information can result from poor-quality data—a situation that gives rise to the expression *garbage in, garbage out. Information* needs to be of high *quality* to be useful.

But what is quality information? In work that remains relevant today, Kahn, Strong, and Wang (2002) noted that IQ was an inexact science in terms of assessment and benchmarks. They advocated for the development of benchmarks to facilitate comparison of IQ across organizations. Another problem is that the terms *data quality* and *IQ* have been used interchangeably (Baškarada & Koronios, 2014). IQ remains a nebulous entity. Everyone believes that he or she knows what it is, but finding a precise, uniformly accepted definition may be an unsolvable issue (Mavetera, Lubbe, & Meyer, 2017). IQ is a multidimensional construct; its dimensions include accuracy, completeness, consistency, objectivity, representation, uniqueness, and timeliness. Not all dimensions are equally amenable to measurement. Objectivity and representation are two dimensions that fall into the difficult-to-measure category (Arazy, Kopak, & Hadar, 2017). Relevance is an attribute that comes up frequently; other criteria may be present, but if the information is not relevant to one's purpose, is it truly quality information (Doering & Maarse, 2015)? A basic description of IQ is effective information that can be used to improve the process of making decisions (Mavetera et al., 2017). Baškarada and Koronios (2014) drew on the classic work of Wang and Strong (1996) and identified 15 dimensions of quality information, which largely reflect many of the attributes identified for data quality. The 15 attributes are:

- Credibility or believability
- Accuracy
- Freedom from bias
- Reputable source
- Beneficial to the task
- Appropriate and useful for the task on hand
- Of an age that it can be appropriate for use
- Sufficient in detail or completeness for the task
- Appropriate in amount
- Clearly defined and in a usable form
- Unambiguous
- Consistent in format to allow comparison
- Compact and concise
- Subject to easy and/or quick retrieval
- Secure

Mavetera et al. (2017) introduced the concept of organization, which is inferred, but not guaranteed, with the discussion of accessibility. That is, when data or information is systematically assembled by a logical scheme, it is easier to find specific items. An illogical scheme or mistakes in assembly can result in very difficult searches. This organization and subsequent presentation of data and information have relevance when one discusses applications of data and its analysis.

◼ Questions to Consider Before Reading On

1. *Discuss what a spreadsheet is, how and where it might be applied in clinical practice.*

2. *What is a database and how is it used? List one database you might use in your practice.*

3. *How are electronic health records (EHRs) utilized?*

4. *What is data mining and how would you apply it in practice?*

◼ Applications of Data

From earlier discussions of the DIKW framework, you have seen how nurses, as knowledge workers, use DIKW during their assessment and care of both individual patients and groups of patients. One can use DIKW without the benefit of computers or digital format, but having data and information in an electronic format provides advantages that include the ability to amass, store, manipulate, share, and reuse data and information much more quickly than can be done without the aid of computers and in larger quantities. Some common examples of data applications that are relevant to support healthcare include spreadsheets, databases, EHRSs, and data mining. Each will be discussed in turn here.

Spreadsheets

A spreadsheet is an electronic document that uses software to display data in rows and columns that can easily be manipulated or used in calculations. A spreadsheet application is typically included in office-productivity software. The spreadsheet application used with Microsoft Office is Excel. Google also provides an online spreadsheet that is free of cost. Common spreadsheet applications include budget preparation and analysis of financial information. Along with the fact that spreadsheets readily support mathematical functions, their ability to organize information into rows and columns also makes them immensely popular for lists of patients and employees, and even in preparing schedules. Spreadsheets also support search functions and allow users to quickly re-order information alphabetically or to increase or decrease values. Spreadsheet files may be generated via manual entries or result from files downloaded from other applications that may include, but are not necessarily limited to:

■ Class lists from learning management systems

■ Missing inventory charges

■ Employee lists generated by human resource or educational software

■ Patient, physician, or provider information from EHRs. Patient-data spreadsheets might include a list of all patients within a specific hospital with a particular diagnosis such as congestive heart failure or an antibiotic-resistant organism, or patients who require wound care.

Spreadsheet files can be visually scanned and/or tallied for use that supports decision making or used as a tool for follow-up. An example of the latter might be a file of all nurses who need to fulfill certain education requirements prior to an accreditation visit (Turnpenny & Beadle-Brown, 2015).

Spreadsheets offer even novice users an easy way to store data and note relationships among different data items. As the volume of data in a spreadsheet grows, reading the data across hundreds of rows and columns becomes tedious, time-consuming, and difficult. When working with large amounts of data that will change and grow, using a database is a more efficient and effective solution. Another aspect to consider is that a spreadsheet only saves the data items or values on the spreadsheet. If a row of data or a single value is deleted from a spreadsheet, the deletion is permanent.

Databases

Databases are software applications that enable the logical storage of many different kinds of data and the creation of various relationships among the data. Data are stored independently of the ways in which it can be displayed, which is one of the major differences between databases and spreadsheets. Another major difference is the search capabilities offered in database software, which enable users to manipulate very large collections of data. Individuals can use off-the-shelf software, such as Microsoft Access, to build databases that can help solve various information-management problems.

The number and types of databases relevant for nurses or that have applications within healthcare delivery is staggering. These include literature databases, various quality measures, and disease-specific databases. Each type is briefly discussed followed by some examples of each. Literature databases allow users to search, download, read, and/or save the latest literature to inform practice. Users can define specific search criteria to limit results returned by date, document type, and whether materials have been subject to peer review. Some well-known examples include PubMed/Medline, CINAHL (Cumulative Index of Nursing and Allied Health Literature), Ovid, and the Cochrane databases.

Many databases collect data for the purpose of demonstrating value or to attain certain predefined measures. The National Database of Nursing Quality Indicators (NDNQI) provides nursing-sensitive indicators that permit the evaluation of nursing care. Nursing-sensitive quality indicators reflect the effect of nursing care on patient outcomes (Mangold & Pearson, 2017). NDNQI was developed by the American Nurses Association as a national database to demonstrate the value of nursing in providing quality patient care (Montalvo, 2007).

The consulting firm of Press Ganey has since acquired NDNQI, which allows it to use evidence of nursing quality with patients' perceptions of their healthcare experience and nurse-engagement data collected through other instruments that they administer (Press Ganey, 2018). Nursing-sensitive indicators represent both structures and processes. Press Ganey partners with healthcare organizations to facilitate understanding of the patient experience. Press Ganey is an independent consulting group responsible for the administration and analysis of patient satisfaction surveys.

The Hospital Consumer Assessment of Healthcare Providers and Systems (CAHPS®) Survey provides a standardized instrument and method to collect data across the nation from patients for the purposes of comparison across providers. The results are publicly reported as an incentive for providers to improve care and increase transparency for consumers. In addition to being publicly available, the results are also reviewed by the Centers for Medicare & Medicaid Services (CMS; Health Services Advisory Group, 2018).

Other databases used to collect hospital data on quality measures include those associated with the Healthcare Cost and Utilization Project (HCUP) and Medicare Provider Analysis and Review (MEDPAR; Agency for Healthcare Research and Quality [AHRQ], 2016). HCUP represents a suite of databases that permit the identification, tracking, and analysis of trends in healthcare use, costs, quality, and patient outcomes. HCUP includes the National (Nationwide) Inpatient Sample (NIS), the HCUP Nationwide Readmissions Database (NRD), Kids' Inpatient Database (KID), Nationwide Emergency Department Sample (NEDS), and NRD, as well as state-specific databases (Agency for Healthcare Research and Quality, 2018). The MEDPAR database contains records on Medicare patients admitted to the hospital (AHRQ, 2016).

Disease-specific databases are used to document variations across all diseases, countries, and cultures to support advances in care. Recently, their focus has been on genomics, otherwise known as *precision medicine*, which provides targeted interventions that are effective based on an individual's genetic makeup (Howard et al., 2012). Some examples of disease-specific databases include:

- Duke Databank for cardiovascular disease
- eDGAR, which is used to collect and organize data on gene and disease associations (Babbi et al., 2017)
- Obesity and Co-morbid Disease Database (OCDD), which was developed to track connections between obesity and comorbid diseases (Ray, Bhattacharya, & De, 2017)
- Orphanet Database, which has information about rare diseases (Pavan et al., 2017)

Electronic Health Record Systems

EHRSs combine the capabilities of database software to collect, store, and manage data and information with other capabilities such as order entry and decision support. When used for planning, delivering, and documenting care for a single patient, EHRSs can expedite timely retrieval of the correct data and information, eliminate issues associated with illegible handwriting, and support standardized terminologies to ensure a uniform meaning to data and information. The result is facilitated communication among healthcare providers caring for a single patient.

The digitalization of patient health records in many healthcare settings facilitates aggregate data collection. Aggregated data can provide evidence for patient-care practices, organizational improvements, and to inform health policy makers. Incentives provided through funds available from the Health Information Technology for Economic and Clinical Health (HITECH) Act and reimbursement monies from the CMS (2017) have helped to make EHRS use in U.S. hospitals nearly universal. Statistics provided by the Office of the National Coordinator for Health Information Technology (2018) showed that 98% of large hospital systems possessed EHR technology as of 2015 with adoption rates among smaller hospitals only slightly behind that number.

Data Mining

Data mining is a relatively new umbrella term or idea encompassing numerous techniques and processes for analyzing very large data sets, with successful results revealing new, valid, and useful patterns (Slimani et al., 2018). As with many emerging concepts, it has numerous definitions and descriptions. Data mining has been described as a scientific field that uses databases, machine learning, pattern recognition, and statistics (analysis and modeling; Brown & White, 2017). When the newly identified patterns are useful in solving problems, data mining has been called a decision-support method. Other experts have added the quality of generating rules for predicting results (Brown & White, 2017). Data mining also has been described as a set of techniques for discovering knowledge (Topaz & Pruinelli, 2017). Most of the analytical methods noted previously are used in data mining.

With the increasing presence of EHRSs and other nursing-related databases, nurses are beginning to conduct their own data-mining activities; however, the number of these studies is still limited. In the meantime, nurses play important roles in this activity. Informatics nurses usually are involved in the information-technology side, conducting the data and information manipulations for analyses. Nurses may serve as data collectors in patient–provider encounters in which the provider is reluctant to use, unable to use, or incorrectly uses electronic data-capture devices. Nurses in this role ensure that clinical data are collected accurately and fully and with standardized terms. Clinical nurses also serve as subject matter experts (SMEs), collaborating on the selection of data items for analysis and consulting on the clinical interpretation of the results.

◼ Questions to Consider Before Reading On

1. *Discuss why it is important to understand how to use data properly. How does the application of data improve practice?*
2. *What is a key component of data analysis?*

◼ Improving Practice

Both data and information are valuable commodities. The ability to use them properly provides multiple benefits that include, but are not limited to, wise use of resources, patient safety, high-quality care, and strategic advantage over competitors (Šilerová, Hennyeyová, Michálek, Kánská, & Jarolímek, 2017). Bringing together data and information from many patients can yield results that address bigger questions or issues such as identifying the impact and effectiveness of selected healthcare treatments while taking into account relevant environmental factors and different causes, symptoms, and patient responses. The steady growth in adoption and use of EHRSs and other digitally based healthcare technologies has resulted in the generation of large amounts of data and information about individual patients. Bringing together (aggregating) the data of many, many patients is creating massive amounts of data, known as *big data* (Brennan & Bakken, 2015).

Data Analysis

Data analysis of massive data sets depends on standardized terminologies. These terminologies include standardized definitions that have meanings that are understood across settings and practitioners. Standardized terminologies support the use of big data because these terminologies enable data to be shared and compared.

Nurses comprise the biggest group of healthcare workers and record the bulk of patient data and information. Big-data analysis of nursing is needed to improve nursing operations, nursing practice, develop informed policies, procedures, and evidence-based practice (EBP) guidelines, synthesize new knowledge, and improve patient outcomes and community health outcomes (Garcia, Caspers, Westra, Pruinelli, & Delaney, 2015). Currently, big-data analytics are difficult to conduct in nursing because nursing information is not captured in ways that make it sharable and comparable (Garcia et al., 2015).

Public-health data and data from EHRs are the first big-data sources usually considered. There are other diverse potential sources for big data in nursing such as clinics, urgent care, schools, insurance claims, laboratories, imaging facilities, social media, and the emerging wearable technologies (Westra & Peterson, 2016). Along with these many sources, there are many types of analyses used with big data. These include—but are not limited to—multiple regression, survival analysis, structural equation modeling, machine learning, social learning analysis, natural language processing, and data mining (Clancy & Gelinas, 2016; Westra et al., 2017; Westra & Peterson, 2016).

CASE SCENARIO

Sue is the infection-control nurse representative for her unit. Currently, the EHRs do not display the presence of drug-resistant infection in a patient's record in a location easily seen or found. Sue receives reports every Friday, which is after many patients have been on the unit for several days or have been discharged. The reports often contain incomplete information.

For example, a prior history of an antibiotic-resistant infection may be noted, but without data on treatment or current status. When Sue complained that the reports as provided are of limited usefulness, the chief nursing officer (CNO) and information technology (IT) staff tell her that she needs to be part of the solution, not part of the problem. Sue would like to have better quality data in a timely fashion.

(continued)

(continued)

Questions Sue Should Explore

1. Can the EHR system provide real-time reports that Sue can run herself and teach other infection-control nurse representatives to do?
2. What factors determine the data that are provided in reports?
3. Where does information on drug-resistant organisms come from?
4. Is there a way to ensure information is communicated among public health offices; community healthcare practices; and acute, subacute, skilled care, and assisted living facilities?
5. What, if anything, can Sue do to improve the quality and timing of reports provided?
6. Is there a way to include information in a manner visible to all staff?
7. How are changes to the system requested, reviewed, approved, and completed?

Questions to Consider Before Reading On

1. *What attributes determine data quality? Information quality?*
2. *Why are data quality and IQ important for nurses? For nursing practice? For healthcare delivery?*
3. *Discuss two causes of data errors. How would you correct these?*
4. *What does information management mean/entail?*

What Can the Nurse Do to Ensure Data Quality? Information Quality?

On an individual level, each nurse has an ethical and professional responsibility to ensure that data that are captured, recorded, and used are of the highest quality and consistent with professional standards of care and practice.

A term often used when discussing the quality of data is *data integrity*. *Data integrity* refers to ensuring the accuracy, completeness, and consistency of data over its life and, as such, is an extremely important concept with information management and the use of software and automated systems. *Information management* is a systematic process that is relevant for all nurses, given that all nurses produce, organize, interpret, and consume data and information in the course of their daily work whether that work is direct patient care, supervision, education, research, or various support activities. The focus of information management is meeting the information needs of healthcare professionals, as well as patients, to support care processes and ensure optimal outcomes. Information management is not a haphazard process. It needs to occur within the framework of a strategy. Maintaining integrity is a key aspect of effective information management strategies. The use of standardized language for uniform understanding is also important for successful information management.

Data and IQ start with accurate and timely data capture, whether that occurs via a manual process or an automated system. In healthcare settings, nurses collect most of the patient data through direct observation or use of various measuring devices (e.g., blood pressure cuff, urinometers, and shift-based patient examinations or assessments). With these manual processes, there always is a time delay between the measurement and the recording of data from the measurement. Time delays increase the chance of errors creeping into recorded data. Simple, human variations among nurses in how they measure a phenomenon and remember the value of the measurement also increase the chance of data errors. Cyganek et al. (2016) noted that human errors in use of electronic records impact the use of that data for analysis. Thus, when nurses are the direct collectors of data, they have a significant responsibility to ensure the quality of the data they collect and document.

When data capture is accomplished primarily through automation, the risk of errors in collection and recording is reduced. This improvement in error reduction is possible only if an automated device is properly designed and regularly tested for quality performance, Software errors (a.k.a. bugs) can generate data errors, so nurses must check the recorded data periodically to see whether they are consistent with an individual patient's trends.

Cyganek et al. (2016) wrote that the data from EHRs are challenging to use for analysis of large sets of data. They noted that the data from EHRs are noisy (i.e., there is a lot of meaningless data), biased, and full of anomalies and gaps.

Nurses can validate that data are accurate and complete at the point of entry. This is accomplished by reviewing selections prior to entry; adding addendums to documentation when required; and, if discrepancies are noted with the capture of biometric data, checking equipment for proper function and/or reporting problems as soon as they are discovered for correction. In the event that nurses note poor quality or erroneous documentation by others, they have an obligation to share their observations and work toward a solution in order to maintain patient safety and quality of care. Solutions may entail working to educate individuals who are not using documentation pathways as intended or reporting problems with the design or limitations of automated documentation for corrective action.

Information management is a term that refers to meeting the information needs of individuals and organizations—something that nurses have a long history of doing through oral reports and nursing documentation. However, *information management* refers to a systematic approach used to ensure that information gets to the people who need it, when they need it, and in the form that they need it. Information management can be considered successful when this process works properly and knowledge and learning occur. Information management in nursing and healthcare includes the following five components:

- An application used to collect, store, retrieve, and analyze data—most often a database such as that seen with an EHR

- A strategy for transforming data into information and knowledge and the systems that process data

- Data
- Systems that support the purpose
- A learning environment that support the previous four components

▨ Questions to Consider Before Reading On

1. *What can the individual nurse do to ensure data quality? Information quality?*
2. *What can nursing, as a profession, do to ensure data quality? Information quality?*

Identify Data-Quality Problems

Nurses rarely see documentation as a priority. Clinical nurses focus on their patients, working to ensure patient safety and patient responses to illness and interventions, and so on. Documenting observations and tasks is a lower priority. With EHRs, documentation is often more timely, due to built-in documentation alerts for planned activities, such as medication administration. Working through multiple screens in an EHR chart while trying to get patient-centered work completed on time can lead to inaccurate or missing data. Thus, the design of data-entry screens and the functionality of the EHR can be a benefit or a detriment.

The absence of standardized nursing terminologies or vocabularies was identified as a data-quality problem earlier in this chapter. Without standardized terms and meanings for those terms, the decisions made based on nursing data can be flawed, potentially leading to poor patient outcomes.

Data Integrity

At its core, *data integrity* means one can trust that the value recorded for a given data item is permanent; it cannot be changed by error or deliberate action of an actor, natural disaster, failure of the storage mechanism and modality, or other factors. In a still relevant article published in 2014, Siegfried Schmitt reported that relatively few instances of data-integrity problems were due to deliberate falsification. The main contributors to these problems were poorly controlled processes for maintaining integrity, poor documentation practices, limited and weak oversight, or even professional ignorance. Schmitt cited work in 2010 by McDowall on naming specific criteria for data integrity. These criteria remain relevant: accurate, attributable, available, complete, consistent, contemporaneous, enduring, legible, original/reliable, and trustworthy. Data integrity provides a foundation for quality information. There are software techniques, referred to as *data cleansing* or *scrubbing*, used to improve the quality of data retrospectively, but the best strategy is to use processes during the initial capture of data that are designed to ensure data integrity. One example of a data-integrity issue is seen when there are different versions of a patient's list of allergies at the family practitioner's office, the hospital's EHR system, and the emergency department's clinical system (Mazzillo et al., 2017; Okafor et al., 2017). This type of problem occurs when there is a mix of manual systems and different electronic systems that do not exchange information. Unfortunately, conflicting or missing data and information can lead to treatment errors and patient harm. Data that are collected, but not shared, are known as a *data silo*.

QSEN SCENARIO

Sue has learned how data, information, information management, and IT are important for patient care and that it is necessary to collecting data in a manner that is amenable to comparison. Structured data, such as that provided through standardized terminologies, seem to be the perfect solution.

1. How would Sue learn more about standardized terminologies?
2. How would she go about selecting and implementing standardized terminology for her clinical area?

Questions to Consider Before Reading On

1. *How do nurses use data? What competencies are needed in order to apply data to clinical practice?*
2. *Discuss four important competencies outlined in AACN (2008) Essential IV. What specifically do these address?*
3. *Why is it important to develop competencies and skills in clinical practice?*

Competency Activities

As knowledge workers, nurses not only collect, record, retrieve, and analyze data and information; they also are consumers of data, information, and knowledge, which they then apply using wisdom. The ability to appropriately apply wisdom, however, requires that the nurse understand the elements involved with the generation and use of data and information. It might be argued that data and information are critical to support each of the nine essentials identified by the AACN for the baccalaureate graduate. *The Essentials of Baccalaureate Education for Professional Nursing Practice* (AACN, 2008, p. 12) states that the baccalaureate graduate should: "Use skills of inquiry, analysis, and information literacy to address practice issues," and "Integrate the knowledge and methods of a variety of disciplines to inform decision making." Essential IV specifically addresses information management and application of patient-care technologies and calls for the graduate prepared at the baccalaureate level to demonstrate the following IT competencies:

- Skillful use to support patient care that includes information systems and communication methods
- Safe practice aided through available tools such as decision support

- Documentation of care that demonstrates attainment of nurse-sensitive outcomes
- Use of standardized terminology to demonstrate nursing's contributions to patient care
- Ability to evaluate data from all sources to inform practice decisions
- Acknowledge the role that IT plays in measuring and improving outcomes
- Maintain ethical and legal standards for the collection, storage, and use of patient data and information
- Appropriate IT use across diverse patient populations
- Recognize the impact of work redesign for patient care and nursing practice
- Ability to evaluate information systems

Nurses prepared at the master's-degree level are expected to serve as leaders, translating evidence into practice and leading change. AACN expects MSN-prepared nurses to demonstrate the knowledge and skills required to provide and coordinate care, using the information technologies of today as well as the evolving information technologies of the future (AACN, 2011). The AACN heightens expectations for nurses prepared at the DNP level (AACN, 2006) to include use of data and information to evaluate outcomes and identify gaps in practice, and to design, select, and use information technologies and information systems.

The QSEN Institute (QSEN, 2018) similarly has identified competencies expected of both the baccalaureate and MSN graduate that reflect many of the same expectations espoused by the AACN. QSEN competencies are divided into the areas of patient-centered care, teamwork, EBP, quality improvement, safety, and informatics. QSEN also calls for ethical practice, a focus on using data and information technologies to measure and enact improvement, and using evidence to inform and support practice. QSEN competencies at the MSN level focus heavily on analysis of data, application of evidence, and the ability to identify strengths and weakness of information systems.

The TIGER Initiative (Technology Informatics Guiding Education Reform), a grassroots effort that originated on the part of nurses as well as more than 70 contributing groups, sought to prepare nurses to use technology and informatics to improve patient-care delivery (Health Information Management Systems Society, 2016). One outgrowth of this initiative was the identification of a list of competencies that every practicing nurse should demonstrate. This list was later operationalized into an instrument for self-assessment of competency levels (Hunter, McGonigle, & Hebda, 2013). Basic computer literacy, clinical information management, and information literacy comprise the knowledge and skill categories identified by TIGER and operationalized in its TANIC (TIGER-based Assessment of Nursing Informatics Competencies) instrument, which remains in use today.

As nursing and healthcare continue to evolve, one can anticipate that new competencies will be identified particularly in areas relevant to DIKW needed to provide safe, patient-centered care. In the interim it is important for all nurses to become adept in the areas identified by professional groups and in government reports.

■ Questions to Consider Before Reading On

1. *What competencies do nurses need to exhibit relevant to data and information?*

2. *Why are the competencies important?*

3. *What should a nurse do to identify and rectify gaps between her or his own knowledge and skills and expected competency levels to apply DIKW and related technologies in practice?*

■ Critical Thinking Questions and Activities

To achieve the recommended informatics competencies for nurses prepared at BSN, MSN, and DNP levels, what are three strategies nurse executives might employ in their organizations?

■ *Which competencies might be the initial focus for each group?*

Now that you have had an opportunity to reflect on Sue's quest to learn more about standardized terminologies and their integration into her clinical area, consider some ways that Sue's nursing colleagues, her organization, and the profession can contribute to this effort.

■ *Give an example of information you can identify that could be improved through the use of standardized terminologies that would add to knowledge about nursing's contributions to patient care.*

SUMMARY

The focus of this chapter has been on the quality of healthcare data and information, with an emphasis on the role and responsibilities of nurses. Definitions and attributes of data and IQ were presented. Ways in which nurses can contribute to the quality of data and information were explained. The chapter included descriptions of the significance of data and IQ for nursing clinical practice, patient outcomes, and the growth of nursing knowledge.

Relationships with the quality of data and information were explored, including (a) information management, (b) the outcomes expected of graduates of nursing programs as identified by the AACN, and (c) competencies expected of the professional nurse as identified by the QSEN project.

■ References

Agency for Healthcare Research and Quality. (2016). *Databases used for hospital quality measures*. Rockville, MD: Author. Retrieved from http://www.ahrq.gov/professionals/quality-patient-safety/talkingquality/create/hospitals/databases.html

Agency for Healthcare Research and Quality. (2018). HCUP databases. Retrieved from www.hcup-us.ahrq.gov/databases.jsp

American Association of Colleges of Nursing. (2006). *The essentials of doctoral education for advanced nursing practice*. Washington, DC: Author. Retrieved from http://www .aacnnursing.org/Portals/42/Publications/DNPEssentials.pdf

American Association of Colleges of Nursing. (2008). *The essentials of baccalaureate education for professional nursing practice*. Washington, DC: Author. Retrieved from http://www .aacnnursing.org/Portals/42/Publications/BaccEssentials08.pdf

American Association of Colleges of Nursing. (2011). *The essentials of master's education in nursing*. Washington, DC: Author. Retrieved from https://www.tnecampus.org/sites/ default/files/docs_and_pdfs/Masters%20Essentials.pdf

Arazy, O., Kopak, R., & Hadar, I. (2017). Heuristic principles and differential judgments in the assessment of information quality. *Journal of the Association for Information Systems*, *18*(5), 403–432.

Babbi, G., Martelli, P. L., Profiti, G., Bovo, S., Savojardo, C., & Casadio, R. (2017). eDGAR: A database of disease-gene associations with annotated relationships among genes. *BMC Genomics*, *18*(Suppl. 5), 554. doi:10.1186/s12864-017-3911-3

Baškarada, S., & Koronios, A. (2014). A critical success factor framework for information quality management. *Information Systems Management*, *31*(4), 276–295.

Brennan, P. F., & Bakken, S. (2015). Nursing needs big data and big data needs nursing. *Journal of Nursing Scholarship*, *47*(5), 477–484. doi:10.1111/jnu.12159

Brown, G. E., & White, E. D. (2017). An investigation of nonparametric data mining techniques for acquisition cost estimating. *Defense Acquisition Research Journal: A Publication of the Defense Acquisition University*, *24*(2), 302. doi:10.22594/dau.16756.24.02

Centers for Medicare & Medicaid Services. (2017). 2017 modified stage 2 program requirements for providers attesting to their state's Medicaid EHR incentive program. Retrieved from https://www.cms.gov/Regulations-and-Guidance/Legislation/EHRIncentivePrograms/ Stage2MedicaidModified_Require.html

Clancy, T., & Gelinas, L. (2016). Knowledge discovery and data mining: Implications for nurse leaders. *Journal of Nursing Administration*, *46*(9), 422–424. doi:10.1097/ NNA.0000000000000369

Cyganek, B., Graña, M., Krawczyk, B., Kasprzak, A., Porwik, P., . . . & Wozniak, M. (2016). A survey of big data issues in electronic health record analysis. *Applied Artificial Intelligence*, *30*(6), 497–520. doi:10.1080/08839514.2016.1193714

Doering, N., & Maarse, H. (2015). The use of publicly available quality information when choosing a hospital or health-care provider: The role of the GP. *Health Expectations*, *18*(6), 2174–2182. doi:10.1111/hex.12187

Garcia, A., Caspers, B., Westra, B., Pruinelli, L., & Delaney, C. (2015). Sharable and comparable data for nursing management. *Nursing Administration Quarterly*, *39*(4), 297–303. doi:10.1097/NAQ.0000000000000120

Health Information Management Systems Society. (2016). History of the TIGER initiative. Retrieved from http://www.himss.org/sites/himssorg/files/TIGER%20History%202017.pdf

Health Services Advisory Group. (2018). The Hospital Consumer Assessment of Healthcare Providers and Systems CAHPS® Hospital Survey. Retrieved from http://www.hcahpsonline .org/

Howard, H. J., Beaudet, A., Gil-da-Silva Lopes, V., Lyne, M., Suthers, G., Van den Akker, P., & . . . Macrae, F. (2012). Disease-specific databases: Why we need them and some recommendations from the Human Variome Project Meeting, May 28, 2011. *American Journal of Medical Genetics. Part A*, *158A*(11), 2763–2766. doi:10.1002/ajmg.a.35392

Hunter, K., McGonigle, D., & Hebda, T. (2013). TIGER-based measurement of nursing informatics competencies: The development and implementation of an online tool for

self-assessment. *Journal of Nursing Education and Practice, 3*(12), 70–80. doi:10.5430/jnep
.v3n12p70

Kahn, B. K., Strong, D. M., & Wang, R. Y. (2002). Information quality benchmarks: Product and service performance. *Communications of the ACM, 45*(4), 184–192. doi:10.1145/505248.506007

Mangold, K., & Pearson, J. (2017). Making sense of nursing-sensitive quality indicators. *Journal for Nurses in Professional Development, 33*(3), 159–160. doi:10.1097/NND.0000000000000323

Mavetera, P., Lubbe, S., & Meyer, J. A. (2017). A student perspective into information quality of web sites. *African Journal of Information Systems, 9*(3), 149–170.

Montalvo, I. (2007, September 30) The National Database of Nursing Quality Indicators (NDNQI). *OJIN: The Online Journal of Issues in Nursing, 12*(3), Manuscript 2. doi:10.3912/OJIN.Vol12No03Man02

The Office of the National Coordinator for Health Information Technology. (2018). Quick stats: Percent of hospitals, by type, that possess certified Health IT. *Health IT Dashboard.* Retrieved from https://dashboard.healthit.gov/quickstats/quickstats.php

Okafor, N., Mazzillo, J., Miller, S., Chambers, K. A., Yusuf, S., . . . & Chathampally, Y. (2017). Improved accuracy and quality of information during emergency department care transitions. *Western Journal of Emergency Medicine, 18*(3), 459–465. doi:10.5811/westjem.2016.12.30858

Pavan, S., Rommel, K., Mateo Marquina, M. E., Höhn, S., Lanneau, V., & Rath, A. (2017). Clinical practice guidelines for rare diseases: The Orphanet database. *Plos ONE, 12*(1), e0170365. doi:10.1371/journal.pone.0170365

Press Ganey. (2018). Nursing quality (NDNQI). Retrieved from http://www.pressganey.com/solutions/clinical-quality/nursing-quality

Quality and Safety Education for Nurses (QSEN). (2018). QSEN Competencies. Retrieved from qsen.org/competencies/pre-licensure-ksas/

Ray, I., Bhattacharya, A., & De, R. K. (2017). OCDD: An obesity and co-morbid disease database. *BioData Mining, 10*, 33. doi:10.1186/s13040-017-0153-5

Schmitt, S. (2014). Data integrity—FDA and global regulatory guidance. *Journal of Validation Technology, 20*(3), 25.

Šilerová, E., Hennyeyová, K., Michálek, R., Kánská, E., & Jarolímek, J. (2017). Influence of the correct management of the IT department on the quality of data and information processing. *Agris On-Line Papers in Economics & Informatics, 9*(4), 91–98. doi:10.7160/aol.2017.090409

Slimani, A., Elouaai, F., Elaachak, L., Yedri, O. B., Bouhorma, M., & Sbert, M. (2018). Learning analytics through serious games: Data mining algorithms for performance measurement and improvement purposes. *International Journal of Emerging Technologies in Learning, 13*(1), 46–64. doi:10.3991/ijet.v13i01.7518

Stausberg, J., Nasseh, D., & Nonnemacher, M. (2015). Measuring data quality: A review of the literature between 2005 and 2013. *Studies in Health Technology and Informatics, 210,* 712–716. doi:10.3233/978-1-61499-512-8-712

Topaz, M., & Pruinelli, L. (2017). Big data and nursing: Implications for the future. *Studies in Health Technology and Informatics, 232,* 165–171. doi:10.3233/978-1-61499-738-2-165

Turnpenny, A., & Beadle-Brown, J. (2015). Use of quality information in decision-making about health and social care services—A systematic review. *Health & Social Care in the Community, 23*(4), 349–361. doi:10.1111/hsc.12133

Wang, R. Y., & Strong, D. M. (1996). Beyond accuracy: What data quality means to data consumers. *Journal of Management Information Systems, 12*(4), 5–34. doi:10.1080/074212 22.1996.11518099

Westra, B., & Peterson, J. (2016). Big data and perioperative nursing. *AORN Journal,* 104, 286–292. doi:10.1016/j.aorn.2016.07.009

Westra, B. L., Sylvia, M., Weinfurter, E. F., Pruinelli, L., Park, J. I., . . . Delaney, C. W. (2017). Big data science: A literature review of nursing research exemplars. *Nursing Outlook, 65*(5), 549–561. doi:10.1016/j.outlook.2016.11.021

CHAPTER 11

ASSESSMENT AND EVALUATING OUTCOMES

CHERYL D. PARKER | MELINDA HERMANNS | CHRISTINE S. GIPSON

LEARNING OBJECTIVES AND OUTCOMES

Upon completion of this chapter, the reader will be able to:

- Explain quality-improvement (QI) methodologies and tools.
- Discuss the concepts of evidence-based practice and informatics skills.
- Compare and contrast QI and evidence-based practice.
- Review how outcome measures apply to quality improvement and evidence-based practice.
- Describe how technology and informatics skills support the process of analyzing outcomes measures.

⊙ KEY NURSING INFORMATICS TERMS

Some of the key concepts and terms you will hear in discussions of healthcare QI and outcomes evaluation are:

Big data

Electronic health record (EHR)

Evidence-based practice (EBP)

Lean

Outcome measures

Outcomes analysis

PDSA—Plan-Do-Study-Act

Quality improvement

Quality and Safety Education for Nurses (QSEN)

Six Sigma

INTRODUCTION: ASSESSMENT AND EVALUATING OUTCOMES

It is imperative for the professional nurse to understand the foundational concepts of nursing informatics—data, information, knowledge, and wisdom are not "owned" by informatics nurses but are part of the practice of every nurse regardless of role. As RNs you know how to collect data and use information to care for your patients. Chapter 13 provides deeper insight into how nurses across the spectrum of care use data and information—from the clinical nurse making decisions about a single patient's care on a given day to the use of big data to support QI and EBP.

▨ Questions to Consider Before Reading On

1. *What do you know about QI, outcomes, and EBP?*
2. *What should you know about these topics?*
3. *How does technology fit in?*

▨ Data Informs Practice . . . or It Should

In the 1970s when making a patient's bed, many nurses were taught when that the pillowcase opening had to be placed away from the door. No rationale or evidence given, just "that is how it is done." Granted, it may look nicer, but other than aesthetics, did it matter?

Much of our knowledge was handed down from generation to generation as experienced nurses taught the novice nurses. Some of these practices seem archaic considering today's evidence. Take, for example, the practice of never telling a patient what medication you are giving to him or he, even if he or she asked! Nurses were to tell the patient to ask the physician about it but to take the medicine anyway. Seems impossible but that was only 40 years ago. The terms *EBP, QI,* and *outcome measures* were not part of the 1970s healthcare culture. Research rarely touched the daily practice of nurses—it was something that happened in a faraway world called *academia.* Fortunately, things have changed.

The early history of research leading to QI included such notable figures as Florence Nightingale,who quantified the relationship between high death rates and poor living conditions, and Ignaz Semmelwiss, who championed handwashing. The road to quality in healthcare delivery has been rocky and achieving quality remains an ongoing effort. According to the Peterson–Kaiser Health System Tracker, the United States lags after comparatively wealthy and developed countries and the gap is widening (Marjoua & Bozic, 2012; The National Academies of Sciences, Engineering, and Medicine, 2018; Sawyer & Gonzales, 2017). This is despite the Centers for Medicare & Medicaid Services (CMS) projections that "under current law, national health spending is projected to grow at an average rate of 5.5 percent per year for 2017-26 and to reach $5.7 trillion by 2026" (CMS, 2018, para. 2).

Ongoing QI is critical for our nation's health—financially as well as for its people. However, you may be asking, what do research, QI, and outcome measures have to do with EBP? And what is the difference among research, EBP, and QI? These are excellent questions.

Ginex (2017) proposed that research, EBP, and QI may overlap somewhat, but there are subtle differences among them. Melnyk, Fineout-Overholt, Stillwell, and Williamson (2010) defined *EBP* as "a problem-solving approach to the delivery of health care that integrates best evidence from studies and patient care data with clinician expertise and patient preferences and values" (p. 51). The U.S. Department of Health and Human Services (HHS & Health Resources & Services Administration, 2011, p. 1) defined *QI* as the "systematic and continuous actions that lead to measurable improvement in health care services and the health status of targeted patient groups" (p. 1). *Research* can be defined as a systematic investigation designed to develop new knowledge, verify current knowledge, or contribute to generalizable knowledge (Ginex, 2017). Outcome measures "reflect the impact of the health care service or intervention on the health status of patients" (Agency for Healthcare Research and Quality [AHRQ], 2011, para. 5). The characteristics of these concepts are summarized in Box 11.1.

BOX 11.1

CHARACTERISTICS OF OUTCOMES MEASURES

TERM	CHARACTERISTICS
EBP	EBP is based on a clinical question. The information gleaned from extensive literature review and analysis of research/patient care data as well as clinical expertise and patient preference and values is used to improve practice. May be done by a single practitioner or an entire health system. Does not have a subject group but is applied to all patients within the defined parameters of the clinical question.
Outcome measures	Measurements that reflect the impact of the healthcare service or intervention on the health status of patients. Can be part of the research, EBP, or QI process.
QI	Does not usually include an extensive literature review and analysis. It is the systematic and continuous actions taken by a healthcare entity that lead to measurable improvement in healthcare services and thereby the health status of targeted patient groups. QI is usually a major undertaking by multiple people.
Research	A systematic investigation designed to develop new knowledge, verify current knowledge, or contribute to generalizable knowledge.

EBP, evidence-based practice; QI, quality improvement.

◼ Questions to Consider Before Reading On

1. *What are the steps of EBP?*
2. *How should EBP fit into daily practice?*

◼ Evidence-Based Practice

In 1972, Archibald Cochrane, a Scottish doctor, wrote a book titled, *Effectiveness and Efficiency*. In it he strongly criticized the common healthcare practices that lacked any basis in reliable research. His work led to the creation of The Cochrane Collaboration, tasked with increasing the number of systematic reviews of research available.

According to Melnyk and Fineout-Overholt (2015), EBP consists of three major components:

1. A systematic search for, and critical appraisal of, the most relevant evidence to answer a clinical question
2. One's own clinical expertise
3. Patient preferences and values

The authors outline seven steps of EBP, numbered 0 to 6:

Step 0: Cultivate a spirit of inquiry.

Step 1: Ask clinical questions using PICOT (population, intervention/indicator, comparison/control, outcome, time) format.

Step 2: Search for the best evidence.

Step 3: Critically appraise the evidence.

Step 4: Integrate the evidence with clinical expertise and patient preferences and values.

Step 5: Evaluate the outcomes of the practice decisions or changes based on evidence.

Step 6: Disseminate EBP results.

It is important to remember that the results that occurred in a controlled research study may not repeat themselves in the everyday practice environment. This is where outcome measures come into play. It is important to monitor the practice change for its impact on patients by measuring the expected outcomes with the results achieved (Box 11.2)

QSEN SCENARIO

Rocio has been asked to develop an EBP project.

1. Where should she start? What informatics skills would Rocio need to successfully complete her project?

BOX 11.2

EXPECTED OUTCOMES MEASURES

Increased	Decreased
Nursing/provider IT technique	Healthcare utilization
Patient IT technique (at least a one-step improvement in technique)	Missed school or work days
All patients receive hands-on teaching	
Asthma control	
Asthma knowledge	
Self-efficacy	
Improved asthma incentive payments	

IT, information technology.

CASE SCENARIO

EXAMPLE OF AN EVIDENCE-BASED PRACTICE PROJECT

Here is an example of an EBP project developed by Gina M. Nickels-Nelson, FNP-BC, MSN, DNP student (2018) at The University of Texas at Tyler—used with her permission. Once asthma rates in Berkshire County, MA, were an ongoing health issue. Berkshire County had the fifth highest emergency room (ER)-usage rates for asthma of all of Massachusetts in 2010. For every 1,000 ER visits, 83 were for asthma.

The City of Pittsfield, Berkshire County, MA, fared even worse. In the City of Pittsfield, MA, 121 of every 1,000 ER visits in 2013 was for asthma. The national average of pediatric asthma in 2015 was 8.4%. In Berkshire County, MA, it was 11.5% and in Pittsfield it was 15.7%.

A review of the literature showed an average of only 40% of pediatric patients knew the correct inhaler technique to use to treat their asthma.

PICOT Question: In pediatric patients with asthma (P), how does hands-on inhaler education (I) compared to verbal-only education (C) affect inhaler technique (IT; 01), follow-up clinic visits for exacerbations (02), ER utilization (03), school attendance (04), and parent work attendance (05) over a 6-month period (T)?

Critical appraisal of the evidence showed:

- Patients do not know how to use an inhaler.
- Verbal education alone is ineffective.
- Family and patients overestimate their ability to use an inhaler.
- Providers and nursing staff do not know how to use inhalers.
- Using an inhaler checklist assesses IT.

QSEN SCENARIO

Given this EBP project, how could Gina measure her project's outcomes?

Questions to Consider Before Reading On

1.   *When considering how EBP fits into clinical practice, what are three barriers to implementing it?*

2.   *What are the steps to implementing EBP into clinical practice?*

Incorporating Evidence-Based Practice

At this point, you may be thinking "this is nice to know but how can evidence-based practice fit into my daily practice?" An excellent question and one needing a bit of background to answer.

In the early part of the 21st century, a new term, *translational research*, began to appear in the nursing literature. The National Institutes of Health (2009) offered the following definition:

Translational research includes two areas of translation. One is the process of applying discoveries generated during research in the laboratory, and in preclinical studies, to the development of trials and studies in humans. The second area of translation concerns research aimed at enhancing the adoption of best practices in the community. Cost-effectiveness of prevention and treatment strategies is also an important part of translational science.

The use of translational research in nursing focuses on the second part of the definition—moving research into practice, that is, EBP. At the time the definition was given, discussions about EBP and the staff nurse centered around improving understanding of and involvement with implementing EBP at the point of care.

But as researchers continued to study the translation of research into practice, several key concepts were documented. Although most studies indicated nurses valued research, the barriers to implementing EBP in their practice cited most often included (Yoder et al., 2014):

- Insufficient time to read and implement research
- Lack of authority to implement needed changes
- Lack of organizational support
- Inadequate infrastructure support such as lack of access to libraries or ethics committees to review research proposals

Many staff nurses, although they value EBP, may see themselves as implementing EBP results with individual patients rather than as active participants in the process (Yoder et al., 2014). You may be thinking you have no skills to be able to critically appraise evidence, so how could you possibly contribute?

As the frontline nurses providing care to patients, we can incorporate the basic steps of EBP into our practice. We can keep up with the latest evidence in our respective specialties, reflect on the current practices in our organizations, question whether those practices are in line with what we are reading, and finally, escalate our concerns if the evidence and practice are not congruent. These four steps are illustrated in Figure 11.1.

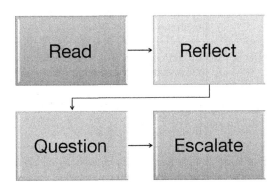

FIGURE 11.1 Steps to incorporating EBP as a frontline RN.

EBP, evidence-based practice.

SOURCE: Copyright 2018 Cheryl D. Parker, PhD, RN-BC, CNE. Used with permission.

Depending on when you last when to school, EBP may not have been part of your studies. But EBP is critical to moving from "we have always done it this way" to a practice culture that questions the status quo. As a member of the front line of patient care, you can participate in EBP committees in your organization, continue to expand your knowledge of EBP process, and perhaps most important, ask why when you see practices that do not align with the latest finding in your specialty area.

Questions to Consider Before Reading On

1. *What are QI methodologies?*
2. *Why is it important for me to know about them?*

Quality-Improvement Methodologies

There are multiple QI methodologies available for use in healthcare and each one has a specific purpose. Box 11.3 provides an overview of 10 commonly used methodologies in healthcare and the basic purpose of each.

BOX 11.3

TEN COMMONLY USED QI METHODOLOGIES

QI METHOD	PURPOSE
1. Clinical audit	Assesses whether a certain aspect of clinical care is meeting recognized standards.
2. Communication tools	Improves quality of care through structured information exchanges.
3. Failure modes and effects analysis	Proactively analyzes all the ways in which a process might fail and eliminates/mitigates the high-priority possibilities.
4. Lean Six Sigma	Finds and eliminates waste in a process. *Waste* is considered any activity not required to provide a service that meets standards.
5. Performance benchmarking	Improves quality by comparing performance metrics to industry leaders, competitors, or best practices.
6. PDSA	Test change on a small scale to see whether change produces the desired improvements.
7. Process mapping	Visually describes the flow of work to identify repetition, delays, and waste.
8. Root cause analysis	Examines the causes of events impacting quality and determines how to avoid them in the future.
9. Six Sigma	Finds and eliminates defects from service delivery using a data-driven approach.
10. Statistical process control	Measures and controls processes quality against predefined parameters.

PDSA, plan-do-study-act; QI, quality improvement.

All nurses should strive to become an expert in the QSEN competencies based on their level of education of QI and informatics (American Nurses Association, 2015; Cronenwett et al., 2007). To be impactful members of a QI project, nurses need to be able to use data, information, and technology to improve patient care.

There are various tools available to support QI methodologies. To see multiple examples, search the Internet ("Images") for the tool.

1. Cause-and-effect diagram (Ishikawa or Fishbone chart): Allows visualization by categorizing the potential causes of a problem so to identify its root causes. It can help identify where and why a process is not working. Assists with sorting out ideas about the problem.

2. Check sheet: A form used to collect and analyze data that can be adapted based on the data needed.

3. Flowchart: A graphical or symbolic representation of a process, including decision points. A swim lane flowchart (or swim lane diagram) shows the process divided visually by who or what is responsible for each step of the process.

4. Gap analysis: This compares the current state with the future/desired state.

5. Histogram: A representation that shows the underlying frequency distribution (shape) of a set of continuous data. Normally, the independent variable is plotted along the horizontal axis and the dependent variable is plotted along the vertical axis.

6. Pareto chart: This contains both a bar and a line chart. In the bar chart, the lengths of the bars represent the important measure, such as time, money, number of errors, complaints, and so on, and is shown on the left vertical axis. The right vertical axis shows the cumulative percentage of the total number of occurrences of the measure represented by the line chart. These are designed so that the longest bar is on the left and the shortest bar is on the right, which allows for a visual representation of the most frequently occurring defects by category. Pareto charts are especially useful in highlighting what is important among a large set of factors.

7. Run charts/Control charts: Run charts are line graphs of data plotted over time to identify patterns or trends. But because a run chart does not use control limits, it cannot show whether the process being measured is stable. Control charts add a central line (average) plus upper and lower control limits to depict how a process changes over time, that is, whether it is stable or fluctuates from the average.

8. Scatter diagram (Scatter plot; Scattergram): Provides a visual representation of the relationship between two variables measured on the same set of subjects.

9. Workflow analysis: A workflow analysis may be used to develop a flowchart of a process. Workflow analysis seeks to understand how the work (process) is occurring so that improvement points can be identified. Technology, such as radio frequency identification (RFID) trackers and wearable cameras, can document movement and help facilitate understanding.

So now that the QI process has occurred, what is next? It would be good to determine whether all our efforts actually made a difference and that we did improve quality. This is where outcomes measures fit into the process.

QSEN SCENARIO

Mark has been asked to participate in a QI project to reduce the number of catheter-associated urinary tract infections (CAUTIs) on his unit. His assignment is to identify gaps between best practice and the current practices on his unit.

1. Where should he start?
2. Where would you start?
3. What QI methods and tools will Mark need to use?

Questions to Consider Before Reading On

1. *What do you know about outcomes measures?*
2. *Why would measuring outcomes be important?*
3. *What is a process measure?*

Outcomes Measures

When you think about any QI initiative, each has one common thread—it relies on data. Descriptive and comparative analytics are widely used in QI. Descriptive analytics analyze retrospective data for patterns to identify what did and did not work. Comparative analytics compare two or more sets of outcomes data—actual outcomes as compared to expected outcomes. The expected outcomes are predefined metrics based on industry-defined key performance indicators (KPIs) and benchmarking, or what research tells us should be the outcomes. Metrics can also be based on a best-guess or gut feeling but that is not a good method, although it is still widely in use in healthcare. Outcomes measures can be used in two ways:

1. Outcomes measures reflect the evaluation of the results of a project and their comparison with the intended results of the project. This means that before starting a QI or EBP project, the outcome measures/expected results need to be determined.

2. Outcomes measures can refer to the measures reported to the CMS for determination of quality care and subsequent payment.

It is beyond the scope of this chapter to discuss outcomes measures and their use in determining payment. We only discuss their use in the EBP and QI process.

In 1966, Donabedian (1996/2005) published a paper titled "Evaluating the Quality of Medical Care," which attempted to evaluate the ways in which quality of the physician–patient interaction was assessed. Donabedian's model proposed a conceptual framework to evaluate quality using three categories:

- Structure: Determines the attributes of settings where care is delivered.
- Process: Determines whether the care that has been provided is appropriate, acceptable, complete, and competent.
- Outcome: Determines the impact of care on patient health status.

The AHRQ uses Donabedian's model to categorize quality measures into three groups (2011):

- Structural measures: These give consumers of health care a sense of the provider's capacity, systems, and processes used to provide high-quality care.

- Process measures: These are steps the provider takes to maintain or improve health, either of healthy people or for those diagnosed with a healthcare condition.

- Outcome measures: These reflect the impact of the healthcare service or intervention provided on the health status of patients.

To account for outside factors, such as differing characteristics within a patient aggregate, statistical models known as *risk-adjustment methods* are used. However, there is debate about the validity of these models. Efforts to refine these models are ongoing.

> **▶AHRQ's Mission**
> . . .to produce evidence to make healthcare safer, higher quality, more accessible, equitable, and affordable, and to work within the U.S. Department of Health and Human Services and with other partners to make sure that the evidence is understood and used.
>
> (www.ahrq.gov/cpi/about/index.html)

There are many types of outcomes data available online. The following lists some types with relevant web addresses. (*Note*: This is not a comprehensive list.)

1. Patient-reported outcomes measures (PROMs) attempt to capture whether the services provided improved patients' health and sense of well-being by asking the patient. PROMIS (Patient-Reported Outcomes Measurement Information System) is available without fee or license at www.healthmeasures.net/index.php

2. The CMS' Hospital Compare rates hospitals based on 57 outcome measures of quality. Information is available at www.medicare.gov/hospitalcompare/search.html

3. County health rankings are available at www.countyhealthrankings.org.

4. The World Health Organization (WHO) Global Health Observatory (GHO) is a data repository that offers statistics on health indicators available at www.who.int/gho/publications/world_health_statistics/2016/en

5. National Center for Veterans Analysis and Statistics develops statistical analyses on topics related to veterans that is available at www.va.gov/vetdata

6. Health Resources & Service Administration—health data by nation, state, and county datawarehouse.hrsa.gov/

If you want to explore all data, statistics, research, and monitoring programs CMS has to offer, go to www.cms.gov/Research-Statistics-Data-and-Systems/Research-Statistics-Data-and-Systems.html

If you really want to immerse yourself in healthcare data, go to www.healthdata.gov where you can find more data sources than you ever thought possible. Not all are open to the public, but many are.

QSEN SCENARIO

Luis has just accepted a position as the only BSN-prepared RN in a primary care clinic in rural western Texas. One of his first assignments is to create an educational pamphlet on diabetes for its patient population.

1. How would the County Health Rankings online database be of use to him?

■ Questions to Consider Before Reading On

1. *A great deal of data are entered into EHRs in today's world, but can it be accessed?*

2. *How are data collected in my organization?*

3. *When would I ever need to analyze data?*

■ Getting and Analyzing the Data

Let us go back to the 1970s again, and think about how health data were acquired for analysis. It was a slow, painful, and expensive process sometimes called *manual data abstraction*. This meant that a person or persons had to manually read through patient charts to pull out the data elements needed. The process was a limiting factor to research in most cases, keeping sample sizes small and time frames to completion long. Imagine spending day after day reading handwritten notes from physicians and nurses to find data elements and then manually transcribing them onto a check sheet. Not only was this tedious work, the chance for transcription errors was always present.

With the widespread adoption of EHRs, technology is replacing manual data abstraction in a variety of scenarios that can improve patient care. EHRs are allowing the analysis of structured health data in volumes impossible to imagine in the 1970s. Instead of a few hundred or even a thousand records, we can now pull data from tens of thousands of patient records.

Natural language processing, the ability for computers to read unstructured text, has been growing in its capacity to abstract data for research. The ability to conduct large-scale population-based research can greatly enhance the efficiency of research efforts.

■ Questions to Consider Before Reading On

1. *What patient data do you document every day?*

2. *How much of that data is useful in making clinical decisions?*

3. *What would help make healthcare data more useful to you in your work?*

> ▶ **HealthPeople.gov Determinants of Health**
>
> The determinants of health are composed of a range of personal, social, economic, and environmental factors that influence health status (HealthyPeople.gov, 2018), such as:
> - Health policy
> - Social factors
> - Health services
> - Individual behavior
> - Biology and genetics

▨ Are We Collecting the Right Data?

Unfortunately, although clinicians document terabytes of data every day, they still may not have access to the data they need at the point of care. Socioeconomic, behavioral, and environmental data, as well as data on the determinants of health, which would allow clinicians to create truly actionable decisions, may not be available at the point of care. The various data elements that make up the determinants of health are found in Box 11.4.

BOX 11.4

DETERMINANTS OF HEALTH AS OUTLINED BY HEALTHYPEOPLE.GOV (2018)

CATEGORIES	DETERMINANTS OF HEALTH FACTORS
Health policymaking	Policies and laws made at local, state, and federal levels impact the health of populations. Examples include banning smoking in public buildings, mandating helmet use when riding two-wheeled vehicles, or allowing construction of a business that produces toxic emissions.
Social factors	This category is broken into two subcategories: social determinants and physical determinants. Social determinants include but are not limited to: • Availability of resources to meet daily needs, such as educational and job opportunities, living wages, or healthful foods • Social norms and attitudes, such as discrimination • Exposure to crime, violence, and social disorder, such as the presence of trash • Social support and social interactions • Exposure to mass media and emerging technologies, such as the Internet or cell phones • Socioeconomic conditions, such as concentrated poverty • Quality schools • Transportation options • Residential segregation Physical determinants include but are not limited to: • Natural environment, such as plants, weather, or climate change • Built environment, such as buildings or transportation • Worksites, schools, and recreational settings • Housing, homes, and neighborhoods • Exposure to toxic substances and other physical hazards • Physical barriers, especially for people with disabilities • Aesthetic elements, such as good lighting, trees, or benches

(continued)

BOX 11.4 (*continued*)

CATEGORIES	DETERMINANTS OF HEALTH FACTORS
Health services	This category includes the barriers to accessing care and the quality of healthcare services available to an individual. Examples of care access include lack of access due to cost, availability, or language issues, whereas quality would include lack of preventive services, treatment delays, or preventable hospital admissions.
Individual behaviors	Healthy or unhealthy behaviors play a significant role in health outcomes. Examples include diet, exercise, and drug usage.
Biology and genetics	Biology and genetics impact some populations more than others. For example, aging impacts health, inherited conditions such as Tay-Sachs, and family health history.

■ Questions to Consider Before Reading On

1. *What patient data do you document every day? What about all the other clinicians working with the same patients you do?*

2. *How much of that data is useful in making clinical decisions?*

3. *What would help make healthcare data more useful to you in your work?*

4. *How would you define big data?*

■ Predictive and Prescriptive Analytics: Helping Us See the Big Picture

What are predictive and prescriptive analytics? Put simply, predictive analytics uses data to predict outcomes, whereas prescriptive analytics goes one step further and suggests actions to take based on the data. Predictive and prescriptive analytics have been around for years and are widely used in today's consumer-buying world. Based on large amounts of purchasing data—yours and other peoples—taken from memberships in store programs, credit cards, online purchases, search histories, and so on, Amazon.com can determine what you would like (predictive analytics) and then recommend those items to you the next time you log on to its site (prescriptive analytics). Google uses similar data and analytics to push targeted ads to your browser. But how would this work in healthcare?

Considering care from a single patient viewpoint, let us look at the Modified Early Warning System (MEWS) tool as an example.

This tool is used by nurses to help monitor their patients with the goal of more quickly identifying patients experiencing a sudden decline in health status. This tool uses six data points—respiratory rate, heart rate, systolic blood pressure, level of consciousness, temperature, and hourly urine output for the previous 2 hours—to alert the nurse of a patient's condition. It would be difficult for an acute care nurse with four to six patients to constantly and consistently calculate these data points by hand, especially given that they are probably located on different tabs or pages in an EHR or a paper-based document.

But this is where the computer has the advantage over humans; it truly can multitask, it does not get bored or distracted, and it will perform the same task repeatedly in exactly the same way every time. If the computer has been instructed to calculate a MEWS score on each of a nurse's six patients every 15 minutes and report whether there have been any changes, it will do exactly that.

But prescriptive analytics takes the next step—it provides the information and then adds recommendations. To make prescriptive analytics useful to direct care providers, there needs to be more data about specific population outcomes that includes the evidence so that specific recommendations and actions can be made for each predicted outcome. For example, if the MEWS not only warned the nurse that the patient data were trending negatively and, based on the patient's age, health history, current medications, and other data, recommended a specific course of action beyond notifying the patient's provider of the change of condition, then we would be moving into the realm of prescriptive analytics.

Keep in mind that prescriptive analytics is not the same as the computer telling us what do to for a patient—just as you determine whether you need to buy something regardless of what the computer recommends—humans have the final say in determining a patient's treatment plan.

▧ Questions to Consider Before Reading On

1. *What actions can you take in the next 6 to 12 months to improve your informatics skill sets?*

2. *How can improving your informatics skills improve your career prospects?*

▧ Big Data—The New Frontier

You might have heard the term *big data* before—healthcare is a producer of big data. *Big data* simply means there are so many data and they are so complex that traditional ways of storing, searching, querying, and updating are not adequate. Chapter 11 is dedicated to helping you learn about big data and its impact on healthcare.

A dashboard of real-time data on patients, including trending and data analysis done by the computer in the background, can help illuminate patterns that humans might miss. Instead of recording and calculating by hand, assessment tools, such as the MEWS, can be calculated and presented to the clinician with visual indicators showing severity.

There are more ways in which you may use data and informatics skills. If you are called on to participate in a unit-based QI or EBP project, what skills can you bring to the table? Skills, such as basic data analysis using common spreadsheet software, can be extremely useful. There are multiple free tutorials online to help you increase your skills.

Understanding the basic structure of a database can also be of value to your career. Free courses are available from Coursera.org and Stanford University.

■ Critical Thinking Questions and Activities

It is important to understand that outcome measures may be affected by many things.

■ *What are some things that can impact an outcome that are outside of the control of an individual or healthcare system?*

Consider a patient you have recently cared for or one you know.

■ *How would having data on his or her determinants of health improve the immediate care of the patient?*

■ *How would having the data impact care planning?*

SUMMARY

Using data and analytics to improve patient care and outcomes, incorporating EBPs, and participating in a QI project are all hallmarks of the present-day RN. These skills do not come from reading one chapter in a book, but from ongoing learning and practice in the real world. Case scenarios reviewing the process of finding and applying evidence into clinical practice were presented. You were challenged with many questions regarding big data and how they are applied in practice and impact care planning. We hope your curiosity has been sparked so that you will be inspired to seek out the next level of learning and experience.

■ References

Agency for Healthcare Research and Quality. (2011). Types of quality measures. Retrieved from http://www.ahrq.gov/professionals/quality-patient-safety/talkingquality/create/types.html

American Nurses Association. (2015). *Nursing informatics: Scope and standards of practice* (2nd ed.). Silver Springs, MD: Nursesbooks.org.

Center for Medicare & Medicaid Services. (2018). NHE fact sheet. Retrieved from https://www.cms.gov/research-statistics-data-and-systems/statistics-trends-and-reports/nationalhealthexpenddata/nhe-fact-sheet.html

Cochrane, A. L. (1972). *Effectiveness and efficiency: Random reflections on health services.* London, UK: Nuffield Provincial Hospitals Trust.

Cronenwett, L., Sherwood, G., Barnsteiner, J., Disch, J., Johnson, J., Mitchell, P., . . . Warren, J. (2007). Quality and Safety Education for Nurses. *Nursing Outlook, 55*(3), 122–131. doi:10.1016/j.outlook.2007.02.006

Donabedian, A. (2005). Evaluating the quality of medical care. *Milbank Quarterly, 83*(4), 691–729. doi:10.1111/j.1468-0009.2005.00397.x (Original work published in 1966 in *The Milbank Memorial Fund Quarterly*)

Ginex, P. K. (2017). The difference between quality improvement, evidence-based practice, and research. *ONS Voice.* Retrieved from https://voice.ons.org/news-and-views/oncology-research-quality-improvement-evidence-based-practice

HealthyPeople.gov. (2018). Determinants of health. Retrieved from https://www.healthypeople.gov/2020/about/foundation-health-measures/Determinants-of-Health

Marjoua, Y., & Bozic, K. J. (2012). Brief history of quality movement in US healthcare. *Current Reviews in Musculoskeletal Medicine, 5*(4), 265–273. doi:10.1007/s12178-012-9137-8

Melnyk, B. M., & Fineout-Overholt, E. (2015). *Evidence-based practice in nursing and healthcare* (3rd ed.). Philadelphia, PA: Wolters Kluwer.

Melnyk, B. M., Fineout-Overholt, E., Stillwell, S. B., & Williamson, K. M. (2010). Evidence-based practice: Step by step: The seven steps of evidence-based practice. *American Journal of Nursing, 110*(1), 51–53. doi:10.1097/01.NAJ.0000366056.06605.d2

The National Academies of Sciences, Engineering, and Medicine. (2018). Announcement: Crossing the quality chasm: The IOM health care quality initiative. Retrieved from http://www.nationalacademies.org/hmd/Global/News%20Announcements/Crossing-the-Quality-Chasm-The-IOM-Health-Care-Quality-Initiative.aspx

National Institutes of Health. (2009). Definitions under subsection 1 (research objectives), section I (funding opportunity description), part II (full text of announcement), of RFA-RM-07-007: Institutional Clinical and Translational Science Award (U54). Available at http://grants.nih.gov/grants/guide/rfa-files/RFA-RM-07-007.html

Sawyer, B., & Gonzales, S. (2017). How does the quality of the U.S. healthcare system compare to other countries? *Peterson–Kaiser Health System Tracker.* Retrieved from https://www.healthsystemtracker.org/chart-collection/quality-u-s-healthcare-system-compare-countries/?_sft_category=quality-of-care#item-start

U.S. Department of Health and Human Services & Health Resources and Services Administration. (2011). Quality improvement. Retrieved from https://www.hrsa.gov/sites/default/files/quality/toolbox/508pdfs/qualityimprovement.pdf

World Health Organization. (1998). Health promotion glossary. Retrieved from http://www.who.int/healthpromotion/about/HPR%20Glossary%201998.pdf

Yoder, L. H., Kirkley, D., McFall, C., Kirksey, K., StalBaum, A. L., & Sellers, D. (2014). CE: Original research staff nurses' use of research to facilitate evidence-based practice. *American Journal of Nursing, 114*(9), 26–37. doi:10.1097/01.NAJ.0000453753.00894.29

PART VI

NURSING INFORMATICS: ETHICS, PRIVACY, AND SECURITY

CHAPTER 12

NURSING INFORMATICS: ETHICS, PRIVACY, SECURITY, OTHER TECHNOLOGY CHALLENGES

CHERYL D. PARKER | CHRISTINE S. GIPSON

LEARNING OBJECTIVES AND OUTCOMES

Upon completion of this chapter, the reader will be able to:

- Discuss the impact technology can have on moral, ethical, and legal concepts in healthcare.
- Explain the differences between *privacy* and *security*.
- Discuss the importance of the difference between professional versus personal social media usage.
- Analyze Health Insurance Portability and Accountability Act (HIPAA) legislation and its impact on nursing practice.
- Analyze current and future technological challenges.

⊙ KEY NURSING INFORMATICS TERMS

Some of the key concepts and terms you will hear in discussions of ethics, privacy, security, and other technology challenges are:

Accountability	Ethical principles
Autonomy	Ethics
Beneficence	Fidelity
Big data	Health Insurance Portability and Accountability Act (HIPAA)
Confidentiality	
Cybersecurity	Internet of Things (IoT)

⊙ **KEY NURSING INFORMATICS TERMS** (*continued*)

Justice	Ransomware
Laws	Security
Morals	Social media
Nonmaleficence	Veracity
Privacy	

INTRODUCTION: ETHICS, PRIVACY, SECURITY, OTHER EMERGING TECHNOLOGIES

Chapter 12 will examine the concepts of ethics, privacy, and security from the perspective of the digital age. With the advent of the Internet of Things (IoT), the pervasiveness of social media, and the expanding use of big data in healthcare, ethics, security, and privacy are more important than ever. From wearable devices monitoring health, to how big data can be ethically used, nurses must gain a more in-depth understanding of how technology is changing healthcare and the challenges that will come with these changes.

▦ Questions to Consider Before Reading On

1. *How well do you understand the similarities and differences of morals, ethics, and law?*

2. *Am I well versed in the professional ethical concepts as set forth by the American Nurses Association?*

3. *How do the concepts of morals, ethics, and law apply to the digital environment?*

▦ Morals, Ethics, and Law in the Digital Healthcare Environment

Before we dive into how morals, ethics, and law apply in our digitally connected environment, let's take a moment to reflect on our past understanding of how these topics apply to us as individuals and in nursing practice.

Ethics is broadly defined as the moral principles of right and wrong that govern a person's decision-making and/or behavior. These principles are guidelines to what is good and bad, right or wrong, that is, decent human conduct. Ethics prescribe what a person ought to do in terms of rights, obligations, benefit to society, and fairness.

The American Nurses Association *Code of Ethics* (2015), simply referred to as The Code, outlines the ethical principles that nurses should adhere to in their professional practice. These principles are justice, beneficence, nonmaleficence, accountability, fidelity, autonomy, and veracity. Box 12.1 provides a simple definition for each principle.

BOX 12.1

ETHICAL PRINCIPLES WITH BRIEF DEFINITIONS

ETHICAL PRINCIPLE	DEFINITIONS
Justice	Persons who are equals should qualify for equal treatment
Beneficence	Do good
Nonmaleficence	Do no harm
Accountability	Respect the uniqueness and dignity of each person
Fidelity	Faithfulness—Displaying loyalty, promise keeping, and respect
Autonomy	Honor the patients' right to make his or her own decisions
Veracity	Be truthful

The Code lays out nine provisions of professional ethical behavior for nurses:

1. The nurse, in all professional relationships, practices with compassion and the recognition of human dignity and worth that is present in every individual.

2. The primary commitment of the nurse is to the patient, whether the patient is defined as an individual, group, or community.

3. The nurse promotes, advocates for, and protects the rights, health, and safety of the patient.

4. The nurse has authority, accountability, and responsibility for nursing practice; makes decisions; and takes action consistent with the obligation to promote health and to provide optimal care.

5. The nurse owes the same duties to self as to others, including the responsibility to promote health and safety, preserve wholeness of character and integrity, maintain competence, and continue personal and professional growth.

6. The nurse, through individual and collective effort, establishes, maintains, and improves the ethical environment of the work setting and conditions of employment that are conducive to safe, quality healthcare.

7. The nurse, in all roles and settings, advances the profession through research and scholarly inquiry, development of professional standards, and the generation of both nursing and health policy.

8. The nurse collaborates with other health professionals and the public to protect human rights, promote health diplomacy, and reduce health disparities.

9. Through its professional organizations, the profession of nursing must collectively articulate nursing values, maintain the integrity of the profession, and integrate principles of social justice into nursing and health policy.

Reflect on this: Are all professional nurses bound by the ANA (2015) *Code of Ethics*?

- Why or why not?
- Can a professional nurse pick and choose which of the nine provisions to apply to her or his practice?

Morals, although similar to ethics, do have some significant differences. Morals may differ between societies and cultures, whereas ethics are generally uniform across all humankind. Morals are the rules or standards of correct behavior made by a society or culture. For example, a given religious society may have rules forbidding its members from receiving particular medical treatments, whereas other religions do not forbid the same treatments.

It is also important to understand the difference between ethics and laws. Ethics are principles or guidelines, laws are accepted rules and regulations. Ethics are more abstract and there are no societal sanctions for violation of ethics unless there is also a violation of a law that is published in writing. Laws are created to help maintain social order and provide protection to the society's citizens. Ethics help people decide what is right or wrong.

Now that we have had a quick review of the concepts of morals, ethics, and laws—let us apply them to the practice of nursing in the digital world and how informatics and technology influence nearly every facet of healthcare.

CASE SCENARIO

John is new on the medical–surgical unit and as such is attending the orientation class on ethics and security for the hospital with other newly hired nurses. They all have reviewed the nine provisions of professional ethical behavior for nurses and taken the quiz offered to demonstrate they understand the information. They are finalizing last processes and moving to the unit to be assigned to a patient care team. John is oriented to the unit, given his security pass code and shown the computers where he will start documenting patient care. He will be sharing this same computer with three other nurses on the unit. He starts his patient care rounds and goes to the computer to start entering information. One of the other newly hired nurses comes up to him and asks that he log in for her as she has forgotten her password.

John starts to consider what he should do:

1. Would it be a security breach to help his peer just this one time?
2. Can he help her document on her patient's chart when he is not caring for that patient? Would this be a privacy violation issue? Are there ethics violations to consider?
3. What is John's responsibility now: to help the other nurse or discuss this issue with his manager? What are John's moral, ethical, and legal responsibilities in this situation?

◾ Questions to Consider Before Reading On

1. *What have the advances in technology brought to the collection of individual health data?*

2. *How is the use of technology-enabled support groups a double-edged sword?*

3. *What are the ethical principles involved in helping educate individuals about their health data?*

Healthcare in the Age of Technology

Advances in technology now allow for data collection and monitoring beyond anything we could have imagined even just 50 years ago. Everywhere you look, people are wearing devices that collect a variety of personal and prescribed data. These devices monitor their cardiac and respiratory functioning, activity levels, blood glucose levels … and the list goes on. Individuals use mobile applications to record their exercise, food intake, and other personal health activities. These devices and applications have the potential to collect real-time data that could help inform research in multiple ways. Unfortunately, relevant ethical practices to guide research in these areas have not kept pace with the explosion of technology (Torous & Nebeker, 2017).

New types of electronically connected support groups have formed using technology platforms, which allow for collecting and analyzing patient data in a completely different way than ever before. These platforms require individuals to create an individual member account and then they are part of the community. Members are free to share their experiences, document efficacy of their medications and treatments, and other healthcare data. These sites may be supported by selling patient-supplied data to pharmaceutical companies, which is clearly outlined in their privacy statements. The massive amounts of unidentified data are shared with the best of intentions; they will help identify unmet needs and generate evidence to improve care. In the mid-2000s, one study announced that a drug under investigation for treating amyotrophic lateral sclerosis (ALS) was ineffectual. However, a patient network site, PatientsLikeMe, announced it had come to a similar conclusion with less cost and sooner than the traditional study (Singer, 2010). These announcements set off a debate about the use of patient-reported data. Critics of this observational method of data gathering pointed to the lack of a placebo control group. Other critics indicated these for-profit networks are primarily interested in making money and their data models lack scientific rigor and that an *N* of 1 or anecdotal data are not valuable (Gorski, 2012).

Ten years later, the idea of patient-generated heath data (PGHD) is a concept that is moving to the forefront of value-based care, which maintains that any and all data about the patient should be valued. The Robert Wood Johnson Foundation funded a joint project with PatientsLikeMe and the National Quality Forum (2017) to "evaluate the novel approach of using online patient-reported data to inform the development and refinement of patient-reported outcome performance measures (PRO-PMs)" (p. 1). The report indicated that patient-reported outcome measures need to be considered in the development of meaningful quality measures.

QSEN SCENARIO

Dolores is a home health nurse caring for Mr. Peters, a 47-year-old Caucasian patient who was recently diagnosed with ALS. Mr. Peters tells Dolores he has joined an online group to connect with other ALS patients. He explains he shares his medication, daily symptoms, responses to treatments, and other personal health data with a community of over 100,000 members.

He is excited about sharing his health data in the hope that it will help others. He also explains he is learning how to better manage his symptoms based on the feedback from others with ALS. He shows Dolores the site and asks her what she thinks about it.

1. What do you know about technology-enabled support groups?
2. What ethical principles would apply in this situation?
3. How should Dolores respond to Mr. Peters' question?

■ Questions to Consider Before Reading On

1. *What are the ethical concerns in the use of social media?*
2. *Can there be any professional use of social media?*
3. *Discuss one ANA principle relevant to social networking. How does this apply to your practice?*

Social Media and Ethical Concerns

Over the last decade, the use of technology and the Internet to communicate information via social networks has increased exponentially (National Council of State Boards of Nursing [NCSBN], 2011). *Social media* is defined as a form of electronic communication (such as social networking websites) through which users share information, ideas, personal messages, and other content (such as photos) in online communities. Social media includes user-generated content on sites such as Facebook, Twitter, LinkedIn, and Instagram (Lachman, 2013; Spector & Kappel, 2012). The use of social media can provide benefits to the nursing profession, but special consideration must be given to the information that is shared online. It is important for the BSN-prepared nurse to understand the difference between professional and personal social media usage.

The NCSBN (2011) published a white paper providing nurses with guidance on the use of social media in a manner that maintains patient privacy and confidentiality while also discussing potential consequences of the misuse of social media. Seven illustrative cases are presented in the white paper that outline actual events reported to boards of nursing (BONs). Nurses can learn about appropriate and inappropriate uses of social media from the analysis included for each case.

The ANA (2011) has developed a document that outlines six principles for social networking as it relates to the nurse. The ANA's Principles for Social Networking state:

1. Nurses must not transmit or place online individually identifiable patient information.

2. Nurses must observe ethically prescribed professional patient–nurse boundaries.

3. Nurses should understand that patients, colleagues, organizations, and employers may view postings.

4. Nurses should take advantage of privacy settings and seek to separate personal and professional information online.

5. Nurses should bring content that could harm a patient's privacy, rights, or welfare to the attention of appropriate authorities.

6. Nurses should participate in developing organizational policies governing online conduct.

The ANA has also developed "Tips to Avoid Problems," which include:

- Remember that standards of professionalism are the same online as in any other circumstance.

- Do not share or post information or photos gained through the nurse–patient relationship.

- Maintain professional boundaries in the use of electronic media. Online contact with patients blurs this boundary.

- Do not make disparaging remarks about patients, employers, or coworkers, even if they are not identified.

- Do not take photos or videos of patients on personal devices, including cell phones.

- Promptly report a breach of confidentiality or privacy.

◼ Questions to Consider Before Reading On

1. *How can we map the health concerns of the United States or the world at a given moment in time?*

2. *Can Twitter be useful in healthcare?*

Tracking Health via Twitter

According to the NowTrending.HHS.gov site: "In March 2012, the Assistant Secretary for Preparedness and Response at the Department of Health and Human Services launched a challenge competition titled Now Trending: #Health in My Community. This contest challenged entrants to create a web-based application that searched open

source Twitter data for health topics and delivered analyses of that data for both a speci-
fied geographic area and the national level." The winners of this contest were two nurses,
Charles Boicey and Brian Norris, as well as a management information systems specialist Mark Silverberg. Their website "Mappy Health" (available at nowtrending.hhs.gov)
became the NowTrending.HHS.gov site.

▧ Questions to Consider Before Reading On

1. *What do you know about security versus privacy?*
2. *Have you given any consideration to your personal privacy and the security of your data?*
3. *How does technology fit in?*

▧ Privacy and Security—What Is the Big Deal?

We often hear the terms *privacy* and *security* and usually consider them interchangeable
terms; they are distinct terms although closely linked. *Security* is defined as "the procedural
and technical measures required (a) to prevent unauthorized access, modification, use, and
dissemination of data stored or processed in a computer system, (b) to prevent any deliberate denial of service, and (c) to protect the system in its entirety from physical harm (Turn &
Ware, 1976, p. 1)." Security is necessary to keep health records from unauthorized access.

Privacy is about people's right to own the data generated about themselves and to control the use of that data. Think back to the first section of this chapter where we learned
about several ways in which patient data can be used. Privacy is the right for each person
to determine how his or her data will be used and who will be able to access, view, or even
share it with others.

Before the days of digital data, privacy seemed a much easier concept: (a) don't let
anyone access a patient's chart unless authorized to do so and (b) be careful where and
with whom you discuss information about a patient. But now the concept of protecting
patient privacy as well as your own is so much more complex.

▧ Questions to Consider Before Reading On

1. *How many HIPAA notifications have you signed since 1996?*
2. *What do you really know about HIPAA?*

HIPAA Basics

We have all signed the HIPAA notification at least a dozen times. But how much do
we really know about it? Health Insurance Portability and Accountability Act of 1996
(HIPAA) is a federal law that sets rules for healthcare providers and health insurance
companies about who can look at and receive a person's health information. Your information can be used for certain purposes not directly related to your care such as state

and federal reporting of population health statistics and as quality reporting measures. Did you know you have the right to ask for a list of everyone who has seen your health information?

The HIPAA Privacy Rule provides federal protection for protected health information (PHI). However, it does allow the disclosure of PHI as needed for patient care and other specific uses.

According to the Summary of the HIPAA Privacy Rule, "individually identifiable health information" is information, including demographic data, which relates to:

> ▶ **Resources:**
>
> HealthIT.gov, "Protecting Your Privacy & Security," available at www.healthit.gov/topic/protecting-your-privacy-security
> HHS.gov, "Your Rights under HIPAA," which includes videos, handouts, and infographics; avaiable at www.hhs.gov/hipaa/for-individuals/guidance-materials-for-consumers/index.html
> Summary of the HIPAA Privacy Rule is available at www.hhs.gov/hipaa/for-professionals/privacy/laws-regulations/index.html

- the individual's past, present, or future physical or mental health or condition
- the provision of healthcare to the individual
- the past, present, or future payment for the provision of healthcare to the individual

Individually identifiable health information is information that can be linked to a specific person or there is a reasonable basis to believe it can be used to identify an individual. Individually identifiable health information includes many common identifiers (e.g., name, address, birth date, Social Security Number). (Taken from www.hhs.gov/hipaa/for-professionals/privacy/laws-regulations/index.html.)

QSEN SCENARIO

Your patient care unit is being remodeled and you have been tasked with making sure the drawers on the new medication carts are HIPAA compliant.

1. What information about the patient can legally be included on the front of the drawer where it can be seen?

Do not guess or use what an employer says—check the HIPAA Privacy Rule—you might be surprised!

Keeping Information Secure—Individual Actions

One way to enhance security is to create strong passwords and to avoid sharing passwords. According to a study by Hassidim et al. (2017), medical staff members often share their passwords with one another in the interest of efficiency. Though it may seem like a good idea to share your password in the interest of time, this is an action that should be avoided to keep information secure.

▶ **Password Security: You Should Care!**
To learn more about managing your passwords, take 10 minutes and visit www.cnet.com/how-to/the-guide-to-password-security-and-why-you-should-care to read a CNET article (CBS Interactive) about passwords.

Creating strong passwords is essential to protecting healthcare data and systems (Venditto, 2015). There are many types of passwords and requirements vary widely among organizations. Some require only letters and numbers, whereas others require a capital letter, special character, and a number, and yet others have different requirements. That said, adding complexity to your password may help defend against certain types of attacks meant to guess your password. According to Cobb (2012), the length of your password is key to improve security and make it more difficult to be hacked. For example, using a passphrase such as "NurseSmithIsARedHeadandwasbornin1982" is a stronger password than "Ps!9@9e" but far easier to remember (Cobb, 2012). Passphrases should be considered when creating a password. The addition of characters to your password increases the number of possible combinations, which makes it more difficult for hackers to guess.

■ Questions to Consider Before Reading On

1. *What is cybersecurity?*
2. *How do you play a role in cybersecurity?*
3. *What is a whaling attack? What is a possible outcome of whaling?*

Keeping Information Secure—Cybersecurity

Cybersecurity is the body of technologies, processes, and practices used to protect the integrity of networks, programs, and data from attack, damage, or unauthorized access. This includes the physical security of the computer hardware as well as protection of the digital data.

When this chapter was written, the major cyberattacks threatening healthcare included ransomware, data breaches, distributed denial of service, business email compromise, and fraud scams. However, by the time you read this chapter, there may be new threats to be aware of—that's how fast technology is changing. Unethical people try to take advantage.

Let us take a quick look at the major cyber threats to healthcare as described by the Center for Internet Security (2018):

■ Ransomware is a type of malware that infects systems and files, rendering them inaccessible until a ransom is paid. Typically, ransomware infects victim machines in one of three ways: (a) through phishing emails containing a malicious attachment, (b) via a user clicking on a malicious link, or (c) by a user viewing an advertisement containing malware.

■ Healthcare data breaches are common and can be caused by many different types of incidents, including credential-stealing malware, an insider who either purposefully or accidentally discloses patient data, or lost laptops or other devices. Personal health information (PHI) is more valuable on the black market than credit card credentials or regular personally identifiable information.

■ A distributed denial of service is an act meant to overwhelm a network to the point of inoperability.

■ In business email scams, scammers use a spoofed email or compromised account to trick employees into initiating a money transfer to an alternate (fraudulent) account. The scammers almost always pretend to be a person of power within the organization, such as the CEO or chief financial officer.

At this point you are probably thinking, I am a nurse taking care of my patients, why should I care about cybersecurity? I do not share my password, we use privacy screens at my work—I am good … right? Well, let us think more critically.

As individuals, we are beginning to keep more and more of our information in digital formats—we communicate by emails and via social media, as well as do our banking and shopping online. As employees, the same is true; email is a primary form of communication, most patient data are online and, if they are not already, they will be in the next few years. Understanding and maintaining your personal security as well as your employer's is critical. Cybercriminals rely on two things: their security-penetration skills and human error … opening an email attachment without thinking or clicking on a link by habit. And what we do not know can hurt us or our employers. For example, did you know that using a URL shortening service could increase the chances that cybercriminals could phish your recipients? Whoops, you do not know what *phishing* is? Box 12.2 provides a list of the most common terms—which are ever changing (Kirchheimer, 2017).

BOX 12.2

COMMON TERMS USED IN CYBER FRAUD TAKEN FROM AARP

TERM	DEFINITIONS
Brute-force attack	A hacking method of finding passwords or encryption keys by trying every possible combination of characters until the correct one is found.
Malvertising	Malicious online advertising that contains malware—software intended to damage or disable computers.
Pharming	This occurs when hackers use malicious programs to route you to their own websites (often using convincing look-alikes of well-known sites), even if you have correctly typed in the address of the site you want to visit.

(continued)

BOX 12.2 (*continued*)

TERM	DEFINITIONS
Phishing	The act of trying to trick you, often by email, into providing sensitive personal data or credit card accounts by a scammer posing as a trusted business or other entity.
Spear-phishing	Phishing that uses personalized email, often appearing to be from someone you know.
Whaling	A phishing attempt on a "big fish" target (typically corporate executives or payroll departments) by a scammer who poses as the organization's CEO, a company attorney, or a vendor to get payments or sensitive information.

Note: See AARP site for full list: www.aarp.org/money/scams-fraud/info-2017/fraud-scam-speak-terminology-guide.html

What can you do to fight cyber crime? Continue to learn about cybersecurity, consider using password protection programs to create and store strong passwords, think before you open an attachment, be careful of what you share online, use up-to-date security software, follow your employer's security polices, and back up your files. Trust your gut: If it seems suspicious it probably is. Did you know that according to a Pew report, 28% of people have not enabled the password or PIN on their mobile devices (Anderson, 2017)? Are you one of the 28%? If so, stop reading and set your passwords now!

As nurses, we understand the importance of patient privacy and security. But in today's digital and interconnected world, we need to expand our thinking to include our own privacy and security as well as that of our employers.

■ Questions to Consider Before Reading On

1. *In what ways are big data collected in healthcare?*
2. *What are the ethical considerations about use of big data in healthcare?*

■ Big Data Is Changing the Game—Ethical Concerns

Big data is exactly what it sounds like—lots and lots of data. How are we collecting healthcare big data? First are the obvious ways such as all the different electronic medical records at healthcare facilities and in provider practices. But another way is the IoT. If you have not heard this term before, think about all the devices in your life that connect to the Internet, collecting and sharing data. Now expand to all the things in the world doing the same—that is the IoT. Devices can now have a level of digital intelligence unthinkable 50 years ago. For example, a pill that knows it has been swallowed and communicates this to a health record.

The concept of the IoT is this: Devices that we would not expect are connected to the Internet and communicating with a remote computer network without any human interaction. Although your personal computer or smartphone aren't considered IoT devices, the smart thermostat in your home would be.

According to Microsoft's (2018) view of the future, IoT solutions will bring multiple benefits to healthcare such as:

- Remote sensors will allow providers to monitor a patient's health status and intervene earlier.
- They will reduce the time spent tracking and managing supplies and medication.
- They will detect problems and repair medical devices before they break.

According to experts, as a society we are lacking frameworks for ethics, governance, and policies in the use of big data and data from the IoT. Technology has no moral or ethical grounding (Berman & Cerf, 2017). The future is going to be a very different place for nursing practice in the next 50 years—as great as the difference between 50 years ago and today.

Questions to Consider Before Reading On

1. *What is the difference between genetics and genomics?*
2. *What are ethical considerations in genomic medicine?*
3. *List one example of robotics. How can it be used in medicine?*

Other Emerging Technologies

Genetics and Genomics in Healthcare

Genetics is the study of inherited traits. Genomics is the branch of molecular biology concerned with the structure, function, evolution, and mapping of genes and sequencing of DNA. It includes the study of the activity of certain genes and their role in specific diseases. The National Human Genome Research Institute (NHGRI; 2016) defines *genomic medicine* as "an emerging medical discipline that involves using genomic information about an individual as part of their clinical care (e.g., for diagnostic or therapeutic decision-making) and the health outcomes and policy implications of that clinical use." Pharmacogenomics involves using an individual's genome to determine whether a particular therapy, or dose of therapy, will be effective.

To put these concepts into a more common framework, genetics will determine whether you carry certain genes, that is, the *BRCA1* and *BRCA2* genes that help determine your inherited cancers risk. Once you have cancer, genomic testing can help predict the aggressiveness of your tumors.

What are some of the ethical considerations of genomic research? The NHGRI (2017) lists the following:

- Possible discrimination by employers or health insurers
- The need for ethical standards for work with human research subjects or tissues
- Consideration of social, cultural, and religious perspectives on genetics and health

Other topics to consider are genetic discrimination, intellectual property, testing regulation, and privacy issues.

Robotics

Robotics is already making headway into healthcare—from surgical robots to nanobots that swim in the bloodstream and deliver targeted medications. Here are several robotic devices we may see in our nursing practice:

- Robear, which can lift patients out of bed into a wheelchair, helps patients stand and turns them (youtu.be/0LaVwDmLDLw)
- Paro the Seal is an interactive "carebot" that moves, coos, and reacts to humans being and is used in dementia (youtu.be/oJq5PQZHU-I)
- Telepresence robots (youtu.be/NfYqQ1TmjNw)

■ Critical Thinking Questions and Activities

Locate nowtrending.hhs.gov/ website on your computer. Reflect on what you learned about how NowTrending.HHS.gov uses data taken from Twitter.

- *Do you think this is ethical?*
- *Once a person chooses to post information about his or her health in a public forum, does he or she lose the right to privacy—why or why not?*

Consider the concepts of morals and ethics in the use of patient-reported data.

- *Which data are valuable and which are not?*
- *Can the patient experience be ignored as anecdotal only?*
- *Are we putting patients and their health information at risk?*
- *How do you think morals and ethical principles apply to selling patient data—even if the sellers have made it clear how the data will be used?*

SUMMARY

In the early 1970s, most hospital rooms were semiprivate and had only one or two electrical outlets. Why? Because the only thing we plugged in at that time was the television. Even the beds had hand cranks. The deluge of technology and the data from those technologies could be better described as a tsunami. And we are in the infancy stage ... think of the very first cars as compared to cars today. The changes will continue to come, and we must be resilient enough to embrace the new models of care. Maybe *Star Trek's* Dr. McCoy was not so far off after all.

This chapter reviewed how ethics, privacy, security, and nursing informatics are relevant and tied together. The ethics of information privacy, security and security issues, and other issues related to the use or incorrect use of technology as well as other technology challenges, including robotics, in today's high-tech healthcare industry were examined. It provided a case scenario and critical thinking questions and activities to consider when applying the concepts laid out in the chapter.

References

American Nurses Association. (2011). ANA's principles for social networking and the nurse: Guidance for registered nurses. Retrieved from https://www.nursingworld.org/~4af4f2/globalassets/docs/ana/ethics/social-networking.pdf

American Nurses Association. (2015). Code of ethics for nurses with interpretive statements. Retrieved from https://www.nursingworld.org/coe-view-only

Anderson, M. (2017). Many smartphone owners don't take steps to secure their devices. Retrieved from http://www.pewresearch.org/fact-tank/2017/03/15/many-smartphone-owners-dont-take-steps-to-secure-their-devices/

Berman, F., & Cerf, V. G. (2017). Social and ethical behavior in the internet of things. *Communications of the ACM, 60*(2), 6–7. doi:10.1145/3036698. Retrieved from https://cacm.acm.org/magazines/2017/2/212443-social-and-ethical-behavior-in-the-internet-of-things/fulltext

Center for Internet Security (CIS). (2018).Retrieved from https://www.cisecurity.org

Cobb, S. (2012). Password handling: Challenges, costs, and current behavior (now with infographic). Retrieved from https://www.welivesecurity.com/2012/12/04/password-handling-challenges-costs-current-behavior-infographic/

Gorski, D. (2012). The perils and pitfalls of "patient-driven" clinical research. Retrieved from https://sciencebasedmedicine.org/the-perils-of-patient-driven-clinical-research/

Hassidim, A., Korach, T., Shreberk-Hassidim, R., Thomaidou, E., Uzefovsky, F., ... Ariely, D. (2017). Prevalence of sharing access credentials in electronic medical records. *Healthcare Informatics Research, 23*(3), 176–182. doi:10.4258/hir.2017.23.3.176

Healthcare IT News (2015). Best practices for password security. https://www.healthcareitnews.com/news/best-practices-password-security

Kirchheimer, S. (2017). Fraud speak—Learn the lingo to beat scammers. *AARP Consumer Protection*. Retrieved from https://www.aarp.org/money/scams-fraud/info-2017/fraud-scam-speak-terminology-guide.html

Lachman, V. D. (2013). Social media: Managing the ethical issues. *MedSurg Nursing, 22*(5), 326–329.

Microsoft Corporation. (2018). IoT for healthcare. Retrieved from https://www.microsoft.com/en-us/internet-of-things/healthcare

National Council of State Boards of Nursing. (2011). White paper: A nurse's guide to the use of social media. Retrieved from https://www.ncsbn.org/Social_Media.pdf

National Human Genome Research Institute. (2016). Genomic medicine and health care (p. 1). Retrieved from https://www.genome.gov/27527652/genomic-medicine-and-health-care/

National Human Genome Research Institute. (2017). Ethical, legal and social issues in genomic medicine. Retrieved from https://www.genome.gov/10001740/ethical-legal-and-social-issues-in-genomic-medicine//issues-in-genetics-genomics-and-health/

National Quality Forum. (2017). Measuring what matters to patients: Innovations in integrating the patient experience into development of meaningful performance measures. Retrieved from http://www.qualityforum.org/Publications/2017/08/Measuring_What_Matters_to _Patients__Innovations_in_Integrating_the_Patient_Experience_into_Development_of _Meaningful_Performance_Measures.aspx

Singer, N. (2010, May 29). When patients meet online, are there side effects? *The New York Times*. Retrieved from http://www.nytimes.com/2010/05/30/business/30stream.html?scp =1&sq=PatientsLikeMe&st=cse

Spector, N., & Kappel, D. (2012). Guidelines for using electronic and social media: The regulatory perspective. *OJIN: The Online Journal of Issues in Nursing, 17*(3), 1. doi:10.3912/ OJIN.Vol17No03Man01

Torous, J., & Nebeker, C. (2017). Navigating ethics in the digital age: Introducing connected and open research ethics (CORE), a tool for researchers and institutional review boards. *Journal of Medical Internet Research, 19*(2), e38. doi:10.2196/jmir.6793

Turn, R., & Ware, W. H. (1976). *Privacy and security issues in information systems*. The RAND Paper Series. Santa Monica, CA: The RAND Corporation. Retrieved from https://www .rand.org/pubs/papers/P5684.html

Venditto, G. (2015). Best practices for password security. *Healthcare IT News*. Retrieved from https://www.healthcareitnews.com/news/best-practices-password-security

PART VII

NURSING INFORMATICS: PROFESSIONAL DEVELOPMENT AND ADVANCEMENT

CHAPTER 13

NURSING INFORMATICS: LIFELONG LEARNING—ADVANCING YOUR OWN EDUCATION

CAROLYN SIPES

LEARNING OBJECTIVES AND OUTCOMES

Upon completion of this chapter, the reader will be able to:

- Determine what professional development is.
- List three areas of professional development. What are some examples of the activities that can be accomplished in each area?
- Discuss why nurses need to continue to develop professionally.
- Discuss the steps in developing a scholarly paper.
- Discuss different software and technology used to develop scholarly works.

⊙ KEY NURSING INFORMATICS TERMS

Some of the key concepts and terms you will hear in this chapter are: The word-processing applications listed below provide the definitions and practical application suggestions for professional practice.

Academics

American Nurses Association (ANA)

American Psychological Association (APA)

Citations

Computer literacy

Electronic health record (EHR)

Grammarly

MASTER (Manuscript Access through Standards for Electronic Records)

Nursing Informatics (NI)

OWL (Online Writing Lab)

⊙ KEY NURSING INFORMATICS TERMS (*continued*)

Plagiarism	Technology
Scholarship	Word-processing software
Spell check	Track changes

INTRODUCTION: PROFESSIONAL DEVELOPMENT

What are some of your experiences with informatics at work and in your nursing program? In the previous chapters, you have learned about hardware and software and how these are necessary for you to complete tasks in your practice. Now it is time to review some applications that can help you further develop your professional skills.

Consider some of the general experiences you have in your current practice environment. What does *professional development* mean? Why is it important in your job role? What is your definition of *NI*? How does your definition tie into what you will learn regarding professional development?

Experiences related to what you may already know from practice and/or have learned from a nursing program will provide the answers to the questions just posed, especially if you have been involved in an EHR implementation. This is where you began to develop informatics skills and the knowledge of what informatics is. These questions may also stimulate your curiosity regarding how informatics skills can be developed if you have not had opportunities to develop them in your practice.

▨ Questions to Consider Before Reading On

1. *What is professional development? How is professional development different from personal development?*

2. *How do you think understanding the processes of professional development might apply to your practice?*

3. *What are some of the NI skills you might use as you continue to develop further in your practice?*

▨ What Is Professional Development?

Professional development using NI skills includes computer literacy, including knowledge of hardware and software functionality and of the practical applications discussed in prior chapters. The focus of this chapter is the application of professional skills development and various word-processing tools to enable you to develop professional, scholarly documents, academic papers, and manuscripts for publication out of the great ideas you will develop.

But what does *professional development* mean? Professional development has several different definitions depending on where it is used. There are two main reasons for skill development—professional development and personal development. The reasons for each type are presented here. You will see they are not necessarily discrete but overlap as personal development can also enhance professional practice opportunities.

Professional development includes earning and maintaining professional practice credentials, such as completing formal courses to achieve an academic degree then attending conferences that offer continuing education (CE) to maintain current practice status. To many, the term *professional development* usually refers to a more formal process such as courses at a university, workshops, or regional conferences. Even if you have completed the primary board licensure and credentials, continuing professional development ensures remaining competent in your practice and should be an ongoing process throughout your practice career.

Examples of professional development expectations from a university are included in Box 13.1.

BOX 13.1

PROFESSIONAL DEVELOPMENT ACTIVITIES

PROFESSIONAL DEVELOPMENT AREAS	ACTIVITIES
Continuing education	• Enrollment in formal degree programs, courses, or workshops • Pursuit of certificates, accreditations, or other credentials through educational programs
Participation in professional organizations	• Attending local, regional, national, and international meetings, conferences, and workshops sponsored by professional organizations • Presenting papers at conferences and workshops • Serving as an officer, board member, or committee member • Coordinating events sponsored by the organization
Research	• Conducting research • Presenting findings of research to others
Improve job performance	• Keeping up with technology, systems, processes • Learning about new developments in your field • Improving existing skills
Improve job performance	• Taking on new challenges in one's current position, projects, long- or short-term assignments

SOURCE: Buffalo State. (2018). Professional development examples, human resource management. Retrieved from https://hr.buffalostate.edu/professional-development-examples.

◼ Questions to Consider Before Reading On

1. *Why do you need to know and understand computer applications to develop professionally?*

2. *Discuss skills needed for lifelong learning; list examples of skills that support lifelong learning.*

3. *What does the acronym MASTER stand for?*

◼ Why Is Professional Development Important?

Whatever the terms, the purpose of professional development is the same. According to Mizell (2010), constant learning can improve understanding of the domains around us as well as afford more and better opportunities to improve one's professional and personal quality of life. Rose's (2018) suggestions of attributes and skills needed for continuous learning—also referred to as *lifelong learning*—include those listed in Box 13.2. Rose developed the MASTER mnemonic to help remember these skills. Mnemonics help us remember what we need to do (Lifelong Learning, 2018).

BOX 13.2

SKILLS NEEDED FOR CONTINUOUS/LIFELONG LEARNING

Motivation	Above all, motivation is critical to lifelong learning; it can come in the form of maintaining an RN license, a performance review, or just being curious about something.
Acquire	*Acquire*, in clinical practice, refers to the integration and development of knowledge to provide safer, quality care for patients.
Search	*Search*, in clinical practice and professional development, refers to the research needed to remain current and relevant in practice. This might be reading an article to support evidence-based practice.
Trigger	A trigger to continuous learning may be an incident at work caring for a patient or some great discussion, performance reviews, or document you reviewed. Whatever the trigger, it serves as a reminder of what you would like or need to do to maintain current practice.
Examine	In professional development and clinical practice you are asked to constantly review what you have learned, how you apply that knowledge, and whether the knowledge is current. If not, you will need to update to current practice through a course or seminar.
Reflect	Many courses you have taken ask you to reflect on what you have learned and how the knowledge applies to your practice. That is the same process used here.

SOURCE: Rose, C. (2018). Master it faster. Retrieved from https://www.skillsyouneed.com/learn/lifelong-learning.html.

Another term often used is *self-directed learning theory*, defined by the educator Malcom Knowles (1975) as:

> *a process in which individuals take the initiative, with or without the help of others, in diagnosing their learning needs, formulating learning goals, identifying human and material resources for learning, choosing and implementing appropriate learning strategies, and evaluating learning outcomes.* (p. 18)

In the second edition of *Nursing Informatics: The Scope and Standards of Practice*, the ANA (2015a) defined Standard 8: Education as "the informatics nurse attains knowledge and competence that reflects current nursing and informatics practice, demonstrates a commitment to lifelong learning through self-reflection and inquiry to address learning and person growth needs" (p. 81) and "integrates nursing science with multiple information and analytical sciences to identify, define, manage, and communicate data, information, knowledge, and wisdom in nursing practice" (ANA, 2015a, p. 2). As discussed in previous chapters, this is accomplished through the use of information structures, information processes, and information technology. These standards are also discussed in Chapter 1.

Because the use of technology is extensive, every aspect of nursing practice falls within the category of responsibility of the informatics nurse, regardless of board certification or not (ANA, 2015a). Regardless of how you achieve leaning, it is imperative to continuous professional development (Bickford, 2015).

▓ Questions to Consider Before Reading On

1. *What is APA style? How would you use it in writing?*

2. *What is OWL? What are some of the topics covered in OWL?*

3. *What is plagiarism? What are some examples of plagiarism? How can it be avoided?*

Resources Commonly Used to Develop Scholarly Works

This section include some tools and resources needed to develop scholarly works for professional growth. The ability to use resources is essential, as is using writing skill as an effective communication tool. Scholarly writing, also known as *academic writing* is writing that clearly and concisely states what has been accomplished, especially when disseminating research that contributes to the advancement of nursing (Morton, 2018). A scholarly paper in nursing needs to follow a strict format that you may already be using, the APA (American Psychological Association) format. According to APA (2010a), *style* refers to the rules and guidelines most publishers and universities require as a standard format used to ensure consistency among documents.

American Psychological Association

There are other citation formats, such as AMA style, used by the American Medical Association (AMA); MLA style (Modern Language Association); and *Chicago* style, developed by the University of Chicago Press. These may be seen in international journals. The style guide most frequently required in nursing is the APA format. As mentioned, when writing a scholarly paper, it needs to follow the strict format outlined in the *Publication Manual of the American Psychological Association*, sixth edition (APA, 2010a), which is the style used in this textbook. What's New in the Sixth Edition of the Publication Manual details the changes in the latest edition (APA, 2010b) There is also an online tool (http://www.apastyle.org → Learning APA Style → Free Tutorials), What's New in the Sixth Edition of the Publication Manual? Free APA Style Tutorials (APA, 2010c). This website provides a quick overview of APA style.

Also, on pages 41 through 59 of the sixth edition (APA, 2010a) of the manual, many sample papers with comments are provided; you will find these samples very helpful when learning the intricacies of the style.

The Online Writing Lab

The Online Writing Lab (OWL) at Purdue University houses writing resources (Box 13.3) and instructional material provided as a free service of the Writing Lab at Purdue. Students, members of the community, and users worldwide will find information to assist with many writing projects. Teachers and trainers may use this material for in-class and out-of-class instruction.

BOX 13.3

OWL WRITING SUPPORT TOPICS

APA style, including the APA Formatting and Style Guide
APA formatting and style guide
ESL
Grammar and mechanics
Job-search writing
Professional writing
Research and citation resources
Subject-specific resources
Tutor resources

APA, American Psychological Association; ESL, English as a second language; OWL, Online Writing Lab.
These can be found at the Purdue OWL website (https://owl.english.purdue.edu).

Citations Versus References

What is the difference between a citation found in the text and a reference? A *reference* is the source you used to find the information relevant to the paper or article you are writing, and the *citation* is its mention in the body of your paper (Sipes, 2018). If you use a direct quote, the quoted material appears within quotation marks and the citation includes the page number on which the quote is found in the original source. A basic example of an in-text quotation follows:

> *According to Sipes (2018, p. xx), "in-text citations need to have quotation marks and a page number."*

Direct quotes longer than 40 words should be placed in block format without quotation marks as in the Knowles quote that appears at the top of page 233. A reference list is added to the end of the paper and includes every source cited in the paper so that it can be located by the reader (APA, 2010a).

Plagiarism Versus Paraphrasing

Paraphrasing refers to expressing someone else's written or verbal communication in your own words; it can help you reconsider the content you just reviewed. Plagiarism, however, is a serious offense and should be avoided at all costs as it can lead to dismissal from school. However, there are many who do not fully understand exactly what *plagiarism* is. More specific, it includes purchasing work developed by others and presenting it as your own, stealing, or "borrowing" work from another source, or even hiring someone to write your paper—all without acknowledging the original source of the material.

In addition, according to OWL (2018), there are also areas of plagiarism that are more difficult to determine. These include using the words of the original source "too closely" rather than paraphrasing them or using others' "spoken or written work" without giving credit to the author (https://owl.purdue.edu/owl/research_and_citation/using_research/avoiding_plagiarism/is_it_plagiarism.htm). Documentation of others' work should also be noted what constitutes plagiarism. In addition to citing quoted and paraphrased material, it is necessary to give credit for tables, figures, diagrams, charts, images from websites, and any other media that you refer to. Also, unless you obtain permission to reproduce such media from the author and publisher, you must recreate that as well. In writing this book all images had to have copyright permission to be reproduced, be omitted, purchased to gain permission for use, or be an original creation.

QSEN SCENARIO

You are beginning to write a paper on an issue you have encountered in your practice but are not sure where to begin.

1. What is a good website you would use that provides guidelines on how to write a paper correctly.
2. What are some of the topics the website covers?

▨ Questions to Consider Before Reading On

1. *List three sources of word-processing software.*
2. *Which software package would you choose? Why?*
3. *What are default settings? Why do you need to set these up?*

◼ Developing a Scholarly Work—Writing the Paper

First you need to decide which word-processing application to use. In Chapter 3, a variety of word-processing applications were discussed: Microsoft Word, Google Drive Docs, and Apple Pages, some of which are commercial products.

Word-Processing Software

There are several free word processors that can be downloaded: Apache OpenOffice: openoffice.apache.org/. Go to OpenOffice.org website → download Apache OpenOffice (2018). Google Docs works with Microsoft Word and PDF files. It also works with other devices, allowing you to create, edit, and share documents from your iPhone, iPad, or Android devices. Use Google Chrome for Mac or PC to be able to work in Docs, even if offline.

Google Docs, Google Sheets, and Google Slides are, respectively, a word-processing program, a spreadsheet program, and a presentation program that all part of a free, web-based software office suite (gsuite.google.com/products/docs) offered by Google within its Google Drive service.

Setting up the Word Processor to Write the Paper

You have decided on a topic for the paper you are writing. As with the previous planning processes you have learned, now you need to develop an outline of what you want to include in the paper. Start with the basic outline and just start writing down some ideas of what you want to say, why you chose this topic, and the impact you might expect the information to have in your clinical practice. You can start by using the word-processing software you selected and find its outline feature, in Word this is Outline View, to create the paper.

- You start by deciding the font and type size to use:12 pt. Times New Roman is standard.
- Next, you will want to define the type of paragraphs indent or block style—and the heading style. Headings are used to organize the material presented. Tops of equal importance use the same heading level.
- If you are using Word, click "View" in the drop-down menu and select "Outline" to set up the format.

You will need to set default settings in the word processor. The default settings are those you set in the software and include APA settings, such as line spacing, required margins, font and paragraph styles, as noted earlier. If writing for a university course, the school will have guidelines you need to follow. There are other settings you can manually set using Word's drop-down menu. Some examples of the options available when creating your document using Microsoft Word follow.

- Select APA style for your citations by selecting "View/Reference Tools/Citations" and selecting "APA" as the citation style.
- Set the indentation and paragraph spacing using the Layout tab (found at the top left of your document).
- To set the margins, choose "Page Setup," also part of the Layout tab.
- Choose "Insert/Table" from the drop-down menu to include tables with numbers of rows and columns, add shapes.
- Add headers, footers, and page numbers by selecting "View/Header and Footer" from the drop-down menu.

Writing the Paper—Putting It All Together

Define the Writing Process

All writing should begin with an idea or issue, something experienced in clinical practice or the review of an article that raises questions, for example. Selecting the topic is the first step. The next step will be a search of the literature—a process described in Chapter 6, with the outline and research information of how and where to start the process of a literature review. The third step is preparing an outline using the word-processing software and setting it up in preparation of writing, starting a draft version to make sure all settings are correct. You will continue to revise your content as you review the material yielded by your literature searches. See Box 13.4 for the steps in the academic writing process.

As you continue a more in-depth literature review, the paper will begin to take form as you focus on the audience you intended and the purpose of the paper. If you hope to publish your paper follow the author guidelines of the intended journal. A great free resource is *Nurse Author & Editor,* an open-access website available to all readers. The advantage of subscribing is that you will receive an email message every time new content is posted on the site (www.nurseauthoreditor.com). There are many other writing resources, including this general resource for helping students learn how to consider writing for professional journals, which is a free web-based course, Writing at the University of Utah, as well as others. Keeping track and documenting the references you want to use is very important when you start writing. Start the reference list to be used at the end of the document.

Tables can be important to include in your document as they can provide a quick summary of key points covered in the discussion sections. Search strategies used to find important information relevant to a topic were covered in Chapter 6 which includes a section on e-literature searches.

BOX 13.4

SUMMARY OF STEPS IN THE WRITING PROCESS

Develop the initial idea, issue, experience, or article to explore.
Conduct a literature search on the chosen topic or topics—then narrow down the topic as you review the literature.
Prepare an outline.
Define your audience.
Define the purpose for the paper.
Document and track needed references.
Start writing the paper by following the outline.

■ Questions to Consider Before Reading On

1. *Discuss the difference between the writing process and writing style.*
2. *Discuss three document basics to understand using APA format.*
3. *Why is a standard process needed to develop a paper?*

A summary of the topic, with page numbers of where they can be found, is included. You should use this worksheet for all papers until you become much more familiar with requirements and how to use the APA manual.

CASE SCENARIO

John is taking a course at the local university and has to develop a paper for an assignment. He has selected two topics of interest to him—bullying and how to find current evidence for best practices—as these are issues he has encountered in his clinical practice. He is searching to find the best evidence to support what he believes is correct practice. John has asked coworkers what their experiences have been when trying to narrow the focus of a topic. He has received many suggestions of the best approach to use for a literature search.

As John continues to have difficulty narrowing the topic down to just one, he begins to search key words: "bullying in the workplace," "evidence-based practice," "best practices" and so on.

(continued)

(continued)

Questions John is exploring with peers:

1. Who else is interested in this topic? The answer will best define his audience.
2. How does it apply to my current work environment and clinical practice?
3. How can I explore both the pros and cons of the two topics, then narrow the topic down further so as to select the one topic?

▨ Questions to Consider Before Reading On

1. After data collection, what should the next step be in the writing process?

2. The paper needs to have different levels of headers. Where can information about this be found?

After developing the outline, the first step in defining the style, other than using APA format, the most common format for nursing writing, is to develop the title. According to the U.S. National Library of Medicine (NLM; 2018), clever or funny titles should be avoided. It is much better to learn to use MeSH (medical subject headings) terms in titles (www.nlm.nih.gov/mesh/MBrowser.html). Using MeSH terminology with links to websites is described in the Chapter 6.

How to pull out all of the different sections of a paper is listed in Box 13.5, with a list of page numbers where guidelines in APA can be found.

BOX 13.5

USING APA TO CREATE DOCUMENTS AND MANUSCRIPTS

DOCUMENT BASICS	PAGE NUMBERS
Title page has appropriate title (no more than 50 characters and spaces); check using word count tool; formatted correctly	229–230
Page numbers	230
Abstract (if required) starts on next page with appropriate header	25–26
Body of paper starts on separate page; the term "Introduction" is not used because it is identified by its position in the paper	229
Headings—Levels 1, 2, 3 (up to 5) are used to separate major sections of a paper; use correct format	pp. 62–63
In-text citations/reference list	174–179

(continued)

BOX 13.5 *(continued)*

DOCUMENT BASICS	PAGE NUMBERS
Summary/Conclusion included	
Reference page starts on a new page; use correct format	37
Write out the word for the numbers 0–9, and any number that begins a sentence; see also section 4.32	111–115
Acronyms and abbreviations; spell out at first use	106–111
Tables (if used) numbered, titled formatted correctly	129
Use spelling ad grammar checks	
Review manuscript for correct format, grammar, citations, reference list	

American Psychological Association. (2010a). *Publication manual of the American Psychological Association* (6th ed.). Washington, DC: Author.

CASE SCENARIO (CONTINUED)

John has had a lot of support from coworkers to narrow and develop a meaningful topic related to his work environment and clinical practice. He is using the worksheet in Box 13.5 as a guide as he beings to develop his paper. He has developed the outline as a guide to follow, created the title page, and now moves toward developing the body of the paper. He was told by peers to always include "Introduction" as a heading on the first page of the body of the paper. It was also suggested that he develop an abstract.

But John believes he has read or heard something different about the way he is to develop the paper and questions what the correct answer might be.

1. Where would John find the information he needs regarding the use of "Introduction" as a header in his paper?
2. Where would he find information regarding when to include an abstract with his paper?
3. After John begins to develop the paper, what are the next sections he will develop after the Introduction?

▣ Questions to Consider Before Reading On

1. *What is the purpose of and how do you use the spell checker?*
2. *How does Track Changes work?*
3. *What is a grammar checker and when would you use it?*

Other Software for Word Processing

In Box 13.5, other tasks were listed that need to be completed before a paper is considered ready for submission in class or for publication. You were asked about a grammar checker and a spell checker. Another frequently used tool in Word is Track Changes, which is especially useful when working with another reader.

Spell checker is a software feature of both Word and Google Docs. It is used to correct spelling errors while using the word-processing program; be careful as the tool may not be correct with the word you are using. To use, select "Tools/Spelling and Grammar" from the drop-down menu. Review tab in the tool bar at the top of your screen—it will open where you will find and click on the Spelling & Grammar icon.

There is a grammar checker, which identifies errors that need to be corrected with a green underline, that is included with the spell checker in Microsoft Word. Tip: Press the F7 function key to start the spelling and grammar checker in Microsoft Word and most word processors. There is also free software available for download known as *Grammarly* (2018). All of these software packages include YouTube tutorials that are very helpful in understanding how to use and apply these tools to your papers (Computer Hope, 2018).

The Track Changes feature, when turned on, indicates where suggested changes have been made in the text and shows comments or questions directed to authors about these changes. If there is more than one additional reader, Track Changes colors can be set to define who said what, for example, Sue's comments are in red, John's in blue. To use this feature in Word, click on the Review tab in the top tool bar of the document, click the Track Changes on/off button and select "Final Showing Markup" on the toolbar and All Markup as well as other functions.

QSEN SCENARIO

In the scenario above, John has completed writing his assignment and is ready to submit it for grading in his nursing course. Before he does that, he remembers there is one last step he needs to complete.

1. How would he check for grammar and spelling errors using Word?

▓ Critical Thinking Questions and Activities

Consider papers you have written in the past.

■ *How would you compare what you wrote then to what you know now about scholarly writing?*

Following the examples shown in this chapter, explain how you would format your next paper by applying the APA guidelines. Develop a sample paper using APA format to create the title, running heads, and body of the text. Include in-text citations, a summary, and a reference list.

You have written this sample paper. Now apply the grammar and spell checkers to that paper. Now review it again using Track Changes to indicate your edits (Study.Com, 2018).

- *What did you find each time you applied the spelling and grammar checkers?*
- *What did you find when another reviewer used Track Changes to edit your paper?*

SUMMARY

This chapter explored professional development and why it and lifelong learning are important to clinical practice. It provided some rationales as to why professional development and continuing education are important, including mandates from national organizations, and how it can impact practice.

The need for nurses to develop informatics skills, including professional development, were discussed based on a number of reports, including the very influential Institute of Medicine (IOM) report. Recommendations to meet these growing needs (IOM, 2010, 2014) require nurses to achieve higher levels of education; this was discussed along with the list of competencies required by many national organizations.

Directions, recommendations, and examples for how to develop scholarly works were provided, including using NI skills and technology to use websites to find important information. Suggestions for using tutorials, such as YouTube, to gain a better understanding of how to use technology, how to use APA style, as well as other resources were included. Critical thinking questions and activities were provided to demonstrate real-life scenarios in application.

References

American Nurses Association. (2015a). Health IT. Retrieved from https://www.nursingworld.org/practice-policy/health-policy/health-it/

American Nurses Association. (2015b). *Scope and standards of practice: Nursing informatics.* Silver Spring, MD: Author.

American Psychological Association. (2010a). *Publication manual of the American Psychological Association* (6th ed.). Washington, DC: Author

American Psychological Association. (2010b). What's new in the sixth edition of the publication manual? Retrieved from http://www.apastyle.org/manual/whats-new.aspx

American Psychological Association. (2010c). What's new in the sixth edition of the publication manual? Free APA style tutorials. Retrieved from http://www.apastyle.org/learn/tutorials/index.aspx

Apache OpenOffice. (2018). Apache OpenOffice. Retrieved from https://openoffice.apache.org

Bickford, C. J. (2015). The specialty of nursing informatics: New scope and standards guide practice. *CIN: Computers, Informatics, Nursing, 33*(4), 129–131. doi:10.1097/CIN.0000000000000150.

Buffalo State. (2018). Professional development examples. Retrieved from https://hr.buffalostate.edu/professional-development-examples

Computer Hope. (2018). What is a grammar checker? Retrieved from https://www.computerhope.com/jargon/g/grammarc.htm

Grammarly. (2018). Grammarly for MS Word and Outlook. Retrieved from https://www.grammarly.com/office-addin

Institute of Medicine. (2010). *Health professions education: A bridge to quality.* Washington, DC: National Academies Press.

Institute of Medicine. (2014). *Keeping patients safe: Transforming the work environment of nurses.* Washington, DC: National Academies Press.

Knowles, M. S. (1975). *Self-directed learning: A guide for learners and teachers* (p. 18). New York, NY: Cambridge Books.

Lifelong Learning. (2018). Skills you need. Retrieved from https://www.skillsyouneed.com/learn/lifelong-learning.html

Mizell, H. (2010). Why professional development matters. Retrieved from www.learningforward.org/advancing/whypdmatters.cfm

Morton, P. G. (2018). Writing for professional journals. Retrieved from https://nursing.utah.edu/journalwriting/

Online Writing Lab (OWL). (2018). Retrieved from https://owl.purdue.edu

Rose, C. (2018). Master it faster. Retrieved from https://www.skillsyouneed.com/learn/lifelong-learning.html

Sipes, C. (2018). Application of Informatics and Technology in Nursing practice; Springer, New York, NY

Study.Com. (2018). What is spell check? Definition and use. Retrieved from https://study.com/academy/lesson/what-is-spell-check-definition-use-quiz.html

U.S. National Library of Medicine, National Institutes of Health. (2018). MeSH keywords. Retrieved from http://www.nlm.nih.gov/mesh/MBrowser.html

INDEX